D0773003

Necrotizing Enterocolitis

Editors

PATRICIA WEI DENNING
AKHIL MAHESHWARI

CLINICS IN PERINATOLOGY

www.perinatology.theclinics.com

Consulting Editor
LUCKY JAIN

March 2013 • Volume 40 • Number 1

ELSEVIER

1600 John F. Kennedy Boulevard • Suite 1800 • Philadelphia, Pennsylvania, 19103-2899

http://www.theclinics.com

CLINICS IN PERINATOLOGY Volume 40, Number 1
March 2013 ISSN 0095-5108, ISBN-13: 978-1-4557-7136-3

Editor: Kerry Holland

Clinics in Perinatology (ISSN 0095-5108) is published quarterly by Elsevier Inc., 360 Park Avenue South, New York, NY 10010-1710. Months of issue are March, June, September, and December. Business and Editorial Offices: 1600 John F. Kennedy Blvd., Ste. 1800, Philadelphia, PA 19103-2899. Customer Service Office: 3251 Riverport Lane, Maryland Heights, MO 63043. Periodicals postage paid at New York, NY and additional mailing offices. Subscription prices are $273.00 per year (US individuals), $401.00 per year (US institutions), $326.00 per year (Canadian individuals), $509.00 per year (Canadian institutions), $400.00 per year (foreign individuals), $509.00 per year (foreign institutions), $129.00 per year (US students), and $186.00 per year (Canadian and foreign students). Foreign air speed delivery is included in all Clinics subscription prices. All prices are subject to change without notice. **POSTMASTER:** Send address changes to *Clinics in Perinatology*, Elsevier Health Sciences Division, Subscription Customer Service, 3251 Riverport Lane, Maryland Heights, MO 63043. **Customer Service: Telephone: 1-800-654-2452** (U.S. and Canada); **1-314-447-8871** (outside U.S. and Canada). **Fax: 1-314-447-8029. E-mail: journalscustomerservice-usa@elsevier.com** (for print support); **journalsonlinesupport-usa@elsevier.com** (for online support).

Reprints. For copies of 100 or more, of articles in this publication, please contact the Commercial Reprints Department, Elsevier Inc., 360 Park Avenue South, New York, NY 10010-1710. Tel. (212) 633-3812; Fax: (212) 482-1935; E-mail: reprints@elsevier.com.

Clinics in Perinatology is also pubilshed in Spanish by McGraw-Hill Interamericana Editores S.A., P.O. Box 5-237, 06500 Mexico D.F., Mexico.

Clinics in Perinatology is covered in *MEDLINE/PubMed (Index Medicus) Current Contents, Excepta Medica, BIOSIS and ISI/BIOMED.*

Printed in the United States of America.

Contributors

CONSULTING EDITOR

LUCKY JAIN, MD, MBA
Richard W. Blumberg Professor and Executive Vice Chairman, Department of Pediatrics; Medical Director, Emory Children's Center, Emory University School of Medicine, Atlanta, Georgia

EDITORS

PATRICIA WEI DENNING, MD
Assistant Professor of Pediatrics, Division of Neonatal-Perinatal Medicine, Department of Pediatrics, Emory University School of Medicine, Atlanta, Georgia

AKHIL MAHESHWARI, MD
Associate Professor of Pediatrics and Pharmacology, Chief, Division of Neonatology, Director, Neonatology Fellowship Program, Director, Center for Neonatal and Pediatric Gastrointestinal Disease, University of Illinois at Chicago, Medical Director, Neonatal Intensive Care Unit and Intermediate Care Nursery, Children's Hospital of University of Illinois, Chicago, Illinois

AUTHORS

NAMASIVAYAM AMBALAVANAN, MD
Professor, Department of Pediatrics; Molecular and Cellular Pathology; Department of Cell, Developmental and Integrative Biology, University of Alabama at Birmingham, Birmingham, Alabama

SACHIN C. AMIN, MD
Division of Neonatology, Department of Pediatrics, Center for Neonatal and Pediatric Gastrointestinal Disease, University of Illinois at Chicago, Chicago, Illinois

VICKIE L. BAER, RN
The Women and Newborns Program, Intermountain Healthcare, Salt Lake City, Ogden, Utah

KATHY Y.Y. CHAN, PhD
Department of Paediatrics, The Chinese University of Hong Kong, Shatin NT, Hong Kong SAR, The People's Republic of China

ROBERT D. CHRISTENSEN, MD
The Women and Newborns Program, Intermountain Healthcare, Salt Lake City, Ogden, Utah

ISABELLE G. DE PLAEN, MD
Associate Professor of Pediatrics, Division of Neonatology, Department of Pediatrics, Children's Hospital of Chicago Research Center, Ann and Robert H. Lurie Children's Hospital of Chicago, Northwestern University Feinberg School of Medicine, Chicago, Illinois

PATRICIA WEI DENNING, MD
Assistant Professor of Pediatrics, Division of Neonatal-Perinatal Medicine, Department of Pediatrics, Emory University School of Medicine, Atlanta, Georgia

PHILLIP V. GORDON, MD
The Division of Neonatology, Department of Pediatrics, Tulane University School of Medicine, New Orleans, Louisiana

MARK LAWRENCE HUDAK, MD
Professor of Pediatrics, Chief, Division of Neonatology, Assistant Dean for Managed Care, Chair, Department of Pediatrics, Associate Medical Director, NICU Wolfson Children's Hospital, University of Florida College of Medicine at Jacksonville, Jacksonville, Florida

HARI IYENGAR, MD
Division of Neonatology, Department of Pediatrics, Center for Neonatal and Pediatric Gastrointestinal Disease, University of Illinois at Chicago, Chicago, Illinois

ZACHARY J. KASTENBERG, MD
Postdoctoral Fellow in the Center for Health Policy and Primary Care and Outcomes Research, The Jack and Marion Euphrat Pediatric Translational Medicine Fellow, Stanford Department of Surgery, Lucile Packard Children's Hospital, Stanford University School of Medicine, Stanford, California

DIANE K. LAMBERT, RN
The Women and Newborns Program, Intermountain Healthcare, Salt Lake City, Ogden, Utah

AKHIL MAHESHWARI, MD
Division of Neonatology, Departments of Pediatrics and Pharmacology, Center for Neonatal and Pediatric Gastrointestinal Disease, University of Illinois at Chicago, Chicago, Illinois

RICHARD S. MANGUS, MD, MS, FACS
Assistant Professor of Surgery, Transplant Division, Department of Surgery, Indiana University School of Medicine, Indianapolis, Indiana

JAMES E. MOORE, MD, PhD
Department of Pediatrics, University of Texas, Southwestern Medical Center, Dallas, Texas

JOSEF NEU, MD
Professor Pediatrics, Division of Neonatology, Department of Pediatrics, University of Florida College of Medicine, Gainesville, Florida

PAK C. NG, MD, FRCPCH
Professor of Paediatrics, Department of Paediatrics, The Chinese University of Hong Kong, Shatin NT, Hong Kong SAR, The People's Republic of China

CLEO PAPPAS, MLIS
Department of Medical Education, Library of Health Sciences, University of Illinois at Chicago, Chicago, Illinois

RAVI MANGAL PATEL, MD
Assistant Professor of Pediatrics, Division of Neonatal-Perinatal Medicine, Department of Pediatrics, Emory University School of Medicine, Atlanta, Georgia

TERENCE C.W. POON, PhD
Department of Paediatrics, The Chinese University of Hong Kong, Shatin NT, Hong Kong SAR, The People's Republic of China

MANIMARAN RAMANI, MD
Assistant Professor, Department of Pediatrics, University of Alabama at Birmingham, Birmingham, Alabama

RENU SHARMA, MD
Professor of Pediatrics, Division of Neonatology, Department of Pediatrics, University of Florida College of Medicine at Jacksonville, Jacksonville, Florida

MICHAEL P. SHERMAN, MD
Professor of Child Health, Division of Neonatology, Women's and Children's Hospital, University of Missouri Health System, University of Missouri, Columbia, Missouri

GIRISH C. SUBBARAO, MD, FAAP
Assistant Professor of Clinical Pediatrics, Department of Pediatrics, Indiana University School of Medicine, Indianapolis, Indiana

KARL G. SYLVESTER, MD
Associate Professor of Surgery and Pediatrics, Hagey Laboratory for Regenerative Medicine, Stanford Department of Surgery, Lucile Packard Children's Hospital, Stanford University School of Medicine, Stanford, California

ROBERTO MURGAS TORRAZZA, MD
Neonatology Fellow, Division of Neonatology, Department of Pediatrics, University of Florida College of Medicine, Gainesville, Florida

Contents

Necrotizing enterocolitis (NEC) is a multifactorial disorder that primarily affects premature infants. Human milk compared with formula reduces the incidence of NEC. Feeding practices do not increase the incidence of NEC in preterm infants. There is no evidence supporting continuous versus intermittent tube feedings in preterm infants. In a feed-intolerant preterm infant without any other clinical and radiologic evidence of NEC, minimal enteral nutrition rather than complete suspension of enteral feeding may be an alternative. Human milk–based fortifier compared with bovine-based fortifier may reduce the incidence of NEC but additional studies are required.

Necrotizing enterocolitis (NEC) is a leading cause of neonatal morbidity and mortality, and preventive therapies that are both effective and safe are urgently needed. Current evidence from therapeutic trials suggests that probiotics are effective in decreasing NEC in preterm infants, and probiotics are currently the most promising therapy for this devastating disease. However, concerns regarding safety and optimal dosing have limited the widespread adoption of routine clinical use of probiotics in preterm infants. This article summarizes the current evidence regarding the use of probiotics, prebiotics, and postbiotics in the preterm infant, including their therapeutic role in preventing NEC.

Necrotizing enterocolitis (NEC) primarily affects premature infants. It is less common in term and late preterm infants. The age of onset is inversely related to the postmenstrual age at birth. In term infants, NEC is commonly associated with congenital heart diseases. NEC has also been associated with other anomalies. More than 85% of all NEC cases occur in very low birth weight infants or in very premature infants. Despite incremental advances in our understanding of the clinical presentation and pathophysiology of NEC, universal prevention of this disease continues to elude us even in the twenty-first century.

Short bowel syndrome (SBS) is the most common cause of intestinal failure in infants. In neonates and young infants, necrotizing enterocolitis, gastroschisis, intestinal atresia, and intestinal malrotation/volvulus are the leading causes of SBS. Following an acute postsurgical phase, the residual gastrointestinal tract adapts with reorganization of the crypt-villus histoarchitecture and functional changes in nutrient absorption and motility. A cohesive, multidisciplinary approach can allow most neonates with SBS to transition to full enteral feeds and achieve normal growth and development. In this article, the clinical features, management, complications, and prognostic factors in SBS are reviewed.

This article is an overview of NEC in term neonates and also summarizes data from 52 cases within Intermountain Healthcare during the last 11 years. In all 52, NEC occurred among neonates already admitted to a neonatal intensive care unit for some other reason; thus, NEC invariably developed as a complication of treatment, not as a primary diagnosis. The authors speculate that the incidence of term NEC can be reduced by identifying neonatal intensive care unit patients at risk for NEC and applying appropriate-volume human milk feeding programs for these patients.

Lactoferrin (LF) is a multifunctional protein and a member of the transferrin family. LF and lysozyme in breast milk kill bacteria. In the stomach, pepsin digests and releases a potent peptide antibiotic called lactoferricin from native LF. The antimicrobial characteristics of LF may facilitate a healthy intestinal microbiome. LF is the major whey in human milk; its highest concentration is in colostrum. This fact highlights early feeding of colostrum and also fresh mature milk as a way to prevent necrotizing enterocolitis.

Current evidence highlights the importance of developing a healthy intestinal microbiota in the neonate. Many aspects that promote health or disease are related to the homeostasis of these intestinal microbiota. Their delicate equilibrium could be strongly influenced by the intervention that physicians perform as part of the medical care of the neonate, especially preterm infants. As awareness of the importance of the development and maintenance of these intestinal flora increase and newer molecular techniques are developed, it will be possible to provide better care of infants with interventions that will have long-lasting effects.

The pathogenesis of necrotizing enterocolitis (NEC) is complex and its speed of progression is variable. To gain understanding of the disease, researchers have examined tissues resected from patients with NEC; however, as these are obtained at late stages of the disease, they do not yield clues about the early pathogenic events leading to NEC. Therefore, animal models are used and have helped identify a role for several mediators of the inflammatory network in NEC. In this article, we discuss the evidence for the role of these inflammatory mediators and conclude with a current unifying hypothesis regarding NEC pathogenesis.

Necrotizing enterocolitis affects up to 10% of neonates who are born weighing less than 1500 g. It has a high rate of morbidity and mortality, and predicting infants who will be affected has so far been unsuccessful. In this article, a number of new methods are discussed from the literature to determine if any currently available techniques may allow for the identification of patients who are at increased risk for developing this potentially lethal disease.

Necrotizing enterocolitis (NEC), a common cause of neonatal morbidity and mortality, is strongly associated with prematurity and typically occurs following initiation of enteral feeds. Mild NEC is adequately treated by cessation of enteral feeding, empiric antibiotics, and supportive care. Approximately 50% of affected infants will develop progressive intestinal necrosis requiring urgent operation. Several surgical techniques have been described, but there is no clear survival benefit for any single operative approach. While debate continues regarding the optimal surgical management for infants with severe NEC, future progress will likely depend on the development of improved diagnostic tools and preventive therapies.

This article summarizes the commonly used biomarkers currently available for diagnosis of necrotizing enterocolitis. The most exciting advances in diagnostic tests were the use of new nucleic acid sequencing techniques (eg, next-generation sequencing) and molecular screening methods (eg, proteomics and microarray analysis) for the discovery of novel biomarkers. The new technology platform coupled with stringent protocols of biomarker discovery and validation would enable neonatologists to study biologic systems at a level never before possible and discover unique biomarkers for specific organ injury and/or disease entity.

> Intestinal failure (IF) occurs when a person's functional intestinal mass is insufficient. Patients with IF are placed on parenteral nutrition (PN) while efforts are made to restore intestinal function through surgical or medical intervention. Patients who fail standard IF therapies may be candidates for intestinal transplantation (IT). Clinical outcomes for IT have improved to make this therapy the standard of care for patients who develop complications of PN. The timing of referral for IT is critical because accumulated complications of PN can render the patient ineligible for IT or can force the patient to await multiorgan transplantation.

PROGRAM OBJECTIVE

The goal of *Clinics in Perinatology* is to keep practicing perinatologists, neonatologists, obstetricians, practicing physicians and residents up to date with current clinical practice in perinatology by providing timely articles reviewing the state of the art in patient care.

TARGET AUDIENCE

Perinatologists, neonatologists, obstetricians, practicing physicians, residents and healthcare professionals who provide patient care utilizing findings from *Clinics in Perinatology*.

LEARNING OBJECTIVES

Upon completion of this activity, participants should be able to:
1. Classify the therapeutic uses of Prebiotics, Probiotics and Postbiotics to preventing Necrotizing Enterocolitis.
2. Explain newer monitoring techniques to determine the risk of Necrotizing Enterocolitis.
3. Describe the use of biomarkers for prediction and diagnosis of Necrotizing Enterocolitis.
4. Discuss Necrotizing Enterocolitis in term infants, intestinal transplantation in infants with intestinal failure, and surgical management of Necrotizing Enterocolitis.

ACCREDITATION

The Elsevier Office of Continuing Medical Education (EOCME) is accredited by the Accreditation Council for Continuing Medical Education (ACCME) to provide continuing medical education for physicians.

The EOCME designates this journal-based CME activity for a maximum of 12 *AMA PRA Category 1 Credit*(s) ™. Physicians should claim only the credit commensurate with the extent of their participation in the activity.

All other health care professionals completing continuing education credit for this activity will be issued a certificate of participation.

DISCLOSURE OF CONFLICTS OF INTEREST

The EOCME assesses conflict of interest with its instructors, faculty, planners, and other individuals who are in a position to control the content of CME activities. All relevant conflicts of interest that are identified are thoroughly vetted by EOCME for fair balance, scientific objectivity, and patient care recommendations. EOCME is committed to providing its learners with CME activities that promote improvements or quality in healthcare and not a specific proprietary business or a commercial interest.

The planning committee, staff, authors and editors listed below have identified no financial relationships or relationships to products or devices they or their spouse/life partner have with commercial interest related to the content of this CME activity:

Namasivayam Ambalavanan, MD; Sachin Amin, MD; Vickie L. Baer, RN; Kathy Y.Y. Chan, PhD; Robert D. Christensen, MD; Nicole Congleton; Patricia W. Denning, MD; Isabelle G. DePlaen, MD; Phillip V. Gordon, MD; Kerry Holland; Mark L. Hudak, MD; Hari Iyengar, MD; Lucky Jain, MD; Zachary J. Kastenberg, MD; Diane K. Lambert, RN; Akhil Maheshwari, MD; Richard S. Mangus, MD; Jill McNair; James Moore, MD, PhD; Palani Murugesan; Pak C. Ng, MD; Cleo Pappas, MLIS; Terrence C.W. Poon, PhD; Manimaran Ramani, MD; Renu Sharma, MD; Michael P. Sherman, MD; Katelynn Steck; Girish C. Subbarao, MD; Karl G. Sylvester, MD; and Roberto M. Torrazza, MD.

The planning committee, staff, authors and editors listed below have identified financial relationships or relationships to products or devices they or their spouse/life partner have with commercial interest related to the content of this CME activity:

Josef Neu, MD is a consultant/advisor for Mead Johnson and Medela.
Ravi M. Patel received a research grant supported by the National Center for Advancing Translation.

UNAPPROVED/OFF-LABEL USE DISCLOSURE

The EOCME requires CME faculty to disclose to the participants:
1. When products or procedures being discussed are off-label, unlabelled, experimental, and/or investigational (not US Food and Drug Administration (FDA) approved); and
2. Any limitations on the information presented, such as data that are preliminary or that represent ongoing research, interim analyses, and/or unsupported opinions. Faculty may discuss information about pharmaceutical agents that is outside of FDA-approved labelling. This information is intended solely for CME and is not intended to promote off-label use of these medications. If you have any questions, contact the medical affairs department of the manufacturer for the most recent prescribing information.

TO ENROLL

To enroll in the *Clinics in Perinatology* Continuing Medical Education program, call customer service at 1-800-654-2452 or sign up online at http://www.theclinics.com/home/cme. The CME program is available to subscribers for an additional annual fee of $212 USD.

METHOD OF PARTICIPATION

In order to claim credit, participants must complete the following:
1. Complete enrolment as indicated above.
2. Read the activity.
3. Complete the CME Test and Evaluation. Participants must achieve a score of 70% on the test. All CME Tests and Evaluations must be completed online.

CME INQUIRIES/SPECIAL NEEDS

For all CME inquiries or special needs, please contact elsevierCME@elsevier.com.

CLINICS IN PERINATOLOGY

DOWNLOAD
Free App!

Review Articles
THE CLINICS

NOW AVAILABLE FOR YOUR iPhone and iPad

Foreword

Necrotizing Enterocolitis Prevention: Art or Science?

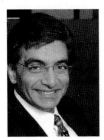

Lucky Jain, MD, MBA
Consulting Editor

It just won't go away!

In spite of concerted efforts by researchers and clinicians everywhere, necrotizing enterocolitis (NEC) continues to be a devastating neonatal illness worldwide.[1,2] Its sudden onset, rapid progression, and ultimate toll on human life are daunting; equally challenging is the lack of any major breakthrough in preventing this ailment. Clinicians treating tiny premature infants live in its fear, jumping at every sign of feeding intolerance and rounding of the abdomen. Clinicians also deal every day with the many stubborn complications of NEC: strictures, short gut syndrome, stunted growth, and poor neurodevelopmental outcomes, to name just a few. For parents, it is perhaps the most disheartening event; after weeks of slow but steady recovery from early complications of prematurity, many or all of the painstaking gains are washed away by a mysterious illness that has no easy cure.

This depressing report card notwithstanding, there have been gains in our understanding of the pathophysiology of NEC.[1] In this issue of the *Clinics in Perinatology*, Drs Maheshwari and Denning have assembled an impressive array of articles highlighting many of these gains; they also point out the gaps in our understanding. The multifactorial etiology of NEC and its varied presentations create a rather complex entity to investigate. The search for better answers continues and we are indebted to this loyal band of investigators and for their persistence.

Yet, there is another aspect of the disease that deserves renewed focus. Why is it that simple measures that can significantly reduce the incidence and severity of disease continue to be ignored[3,4]? For example, neonatal intensive care units (NICUs) with exclusive use of breast milk for preterm infants report a strikingly lower incidence of NEC.[5] A recent quality improvement project in California to increase breast milk use in very low birth weight infants resulted in a reduction of NEC from 7% to 2.4%.[5]

Clin Perinatol 40 (2013) xiii–xv
http://dx.doi.org/10.1016/j.clp.2013.01.002
0095-5108/13/$ – see front matter © 2013 Published by Elsevier Inc.

Numerous other studies have shown similar results in the past.[4] Yet, discussions with parents seldom include objective evidence and data about the benefits of breast milk. Hospitals suffer from a chronic shortage of qualified lactation consultants and few have access to donor milk. The result: an unacceptably low rate of breast milk feeds for our most vulnerable patients.

There is also the conundrum of how we should feed our tiny premature infants. Few NICUs use standardized protocols, making it impossible to tell which practice does more harm than good. Huge practice variations exist in when feeds are started, how they are advanced, and how feeding intolerance is managed.[2] There is a growing trend toward transpyloric feeds and acid suppression, strategies that potentially encourage bacterial overgrowth and predisposition to sepsis.

There is a growing interest in the microbial ecosystem of the human intestine and the vital role it can play in protecting the host against disease.[6] Probiotics and prebiotics are currently being tested in several clinical trials. It is possible that positive results from these trials will help bring them into our clinical armamentarium and help standardize the proper regimen of probiotics to be used. Yet, little attention is paid to the natural microbiome with which each newborn starts. There are distinct differences in the microbiome of children born by cesarean section compared to those delivered vaginally. Similar differences exist in newborns who receive even the shortest courses of antibiotics to "rule out sepsis." The neonatal community is yet to embrace a uniform approach to managing these simple issues and strategies that would reduce the cumulative exposure of newborns to antibiotics.

Given all these differences in practice styles, it should come as no surprise that the rates of NEC vary widely among centers. While basic science and translational research continue the quest to find the next magic bullet, does it not make sense for us to start with best practices that have already been shown to make a difference?

We hope that this issue of the *Clinics in Perinatology* will stimulate discussion about these many aspects of this complex disease. Drs Maheshwari and Denning are to be congratulated for putting together a remarkable set of articles by thought leaders in the field. I am also grateful to Kerry Holland and Elsevier for their support. Our hospital now proudly tracks months elapsed without a central line–associated bloodstream infection (**Fig. 1**). I am waiting for the day when we start doing the same for NEC!

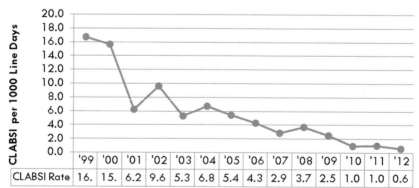

EG NICU CLABSI Rate

	'99	'00	'01	'02	'03	'04	'05	'06	'07	'08	'09	'10	'11	'12
CLABSI Rate	16.	15.	6.2	9.6	5.3	6.8	5.4	4.3	2.9	3.7	2.5	1.0	1.0	0.6

Fig. 1. Experience over time with central line–associated bloodstream infections (CLABSI) at a single institution from 1999 to 2012. EG, Egleston. (*Unpublished data, Courtesy of* Children's Healthcare of Atlanta NICU Team.)

Lucky Jain, MD, MBA
Department of Pediatrics, Emory Children's Center
Emory University School of Medicine
2015 Uppergate Drive
Atlanta, GA 30322, USA

E-mail address:
ljain@emory.edu

REFERENCES

1. Neu J, Walker WA. Necrotizing enterocolitis. N Engl J Med 2011;364:255–64.
2. Athalye-Jape G, More K, Patole S. Progress in the field of necrotizing enterocolitis— year 2012. J Matern Fetal Neonatal Med 2012;1–8 [Epub ahead of print].
3. Swanson J. Necrotizing enterocolitis: is it time for zero tolerance? J Perinatol 2013; 33:1–2.
4. Underwood MA. Human milk for the premature infant. Pediatr Clin North Am 2013; 60:189–207.
5. Lee HC, Kurtin PS, Wight NE, et al. A quality improvement project to increase breast milk use in very low birth weight infants. Pediatrics 2012;130:e1679–87.
6. Audy EO, Claud EC, Gloor GB, et al. Microbial ecosystems therapeutics: a new paradigm in medicine? Benef Microbes 2012;20:1–13.

Preface

Necrotizing Enterocolitis: Hope on the Horizon

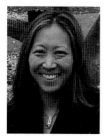 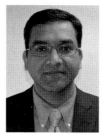

Patricia Wei Denning, MD   Akhil Maheshwari, MD
Editors

At long last, we are finally making progress in our understanding of necrotizing entero-colitis (NEC). As the readership of this periodical is well aware, despite all the successes of neonatal intensive care, the mortality and morbidity of NEC have re-mained largely unchanged. However, the past decade has seen new ground being broken in all areas of NEC research, including early diagnosis, medical and surgical management of acute NEC, and rehabilitation of those with a complicated disease course.

NEC is one of the few diseases that we still diagnose based on radiologic and/or histopathologic findings. Needless to say, by the time characteristic radiologic findings of unrestricted bacterial overgrowth such as pneumatosis, or those of peritonitis such as fixed bowel loops and ascites, are detected, or if the patient is already at a stage where histopathology is available as a diagnostic option (the infant has already had a visit to the operating room), it may be a bit too late for an "intestine-saving" interven-tion. The lack of early-stage biomarkers has also limited our ability to enroll patients into clinical trials of new treatments at a stage when tissue can still be saved, the systemic inflammatory response can still be prevented, and yet be certain that the patient actually has NEC and not feeding intolerance due to immaturity or an alternative cause such as septic ileus.

NEC is also one of the few diseases that derive their description from characteristic histopathologic findings. Epidemiologically, the risk factors may originate in utero, such as chorioamnionitis and placental insufficiency; at the time of birth, such as peri-natal asphyxia; or later, such as indomethacin therapy, viral infections, and blood

Clin Perinatol 40 (2013) xvii–xix
http://dx.doi.org/10.1016/j.clp.2013.01.001
0095-5108/13/$ – see front matter © 2013 Published by Elsevier Inc.   **perinatology.theclinics.com**

transfusions. Such diversity of risk factors is by no means unique to NEC and may possibly be the case with every condition that derives its identity in its pathoanatomy, such as cirrhosis of the liver, where viruses, alcohol, and toxins can all lead to the same histoarchitectural change. NEC, which is defined by the presence of coagulative necrosis, bacterial overgrowth, pneumatosis, and a cellular inflammatory response (**Fig. 1**), may also represent a situation where the pathoanatomy points not to a single etiologic pathway but may instead represent a generic tissue injury response of the gastrointestinal tract at a specific stage of development. Philosophically, this realization can help in shaping our expectations—if NEC is indeed a group of several distinct nosologic entities, treatment efforts may need to be tailored to each subgroup. We may also have to accept that we may never eliminate NEC completely—as we control today's causes of NEC, it is possible that new causes will appear in time as our patient population and practices change.

In this issue of the *Clinics in Perinatology*, our attempt has been to focus on some of the major dilemmas that all of us face in the neonatal intensive care unit. We hope that you will enjoy the articles by Drs Ambalavanan and Ramani, Sharma and Hudak, and Christensen on the role of feeding, clinical presentations of NEC, and the changing face of NEC in full-term neonates, respectively. The articles on gut microbiome and inflammatory signaling by Drs Neu and DePlaen summarize the current state of the science in the laboratory. Drs Sherman, Moore, and Ng, Chan, and Poon bring us authoritative descriptions of some of the most exciting developments in this field. Our own groups have contributed articles on short bowel syndrome and probiotics, and finally, Drs Mangus and Subbarao bring you everything you ever wanted to know (but were afraid to ask) about intestinal transplantation.

We wish to thank Dr Lucky Jain for his encouragement in bringing out this volume; Kerry Holland, Senior Editor, for all her support; and Nicole Congleton, for editorial assistance. We, of course, are indebted to and grateful to the authors whose contributions will be fully appreciated by the readers, and to our families (Ritu, Jayant, and

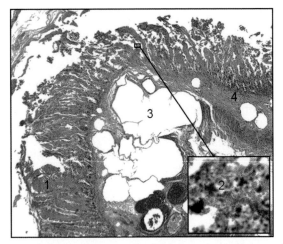

Fig. 1. Photomicrograph from a hematoxylin & eosin–stained tissue section of NEC. The diagnosis of NEC rests on the detection of characteristic histopathologic features: coagulative necrosis (1), bacterial overgrowth (2), pneumatosis (3), and a cellular inflammatory response (4).

Vikram; and Tim, Christopher, Connor, Mia, Brianna, and Adia) for their enduring support.

Patricia Wei Denning, MD
Division of Neonatal-Perinatal Medicine
Department of Pediatrics
Emory University School of Medicine
2015 Uppergate Drive
Atlanta, GA 30322, USA

Akhil Maheshwari, MD
University of Illinois at Chicago
840 South Wood Street, CSB 1257
Chicago, IL 60612, USA

E-mail addresses:
pllin@emory.edu (P.W. Denning)
akhil1@uic.edu (A. Maheshwari)

Feeding Practices and Necrotizing Enterocolitis

Manimaran Ramani, MD[a], Namasivayam Ambalavanan, MD[a,b,c],*

KEYWORDS

- Necrotizing enterocolitis • Feeding methods • Enteral nutrition • Premature infant

KEY POINTS

- The evidence is convincing that human milk feeding, compared with formula feeding, reduces the incidence of necrotizing enterocolitis (NEC) in preterm infants.
- Minimal enteral nutrition (MEN) is a safe alternative to complete fasting before initiation of progressive feedings and does not increase the incidence of NEC in extremely preterm infants. In clinically stable very low-birth-weight (VLBW) infants, early introduction of progressive feeds and advancement of feeds at a faster rate (30–35 mL/kg/d) is safe and does not increase the incidence of NEC.
- There is no evidence supporting continuous versus intermittent tube feedings in preterm infants.
- In a feed-intolerant preterm infant without any other clinical and radiologic evidence of NEC, MEN rather than complete suspension of enteral feeding may be an alternative.
- Human milk-based fortifier compared with bovine-based fortifier may reduce the incidence of NEC but additional studies are required.

INTRODUCTION

NEC is an acute ischemic necrotizing disease of the gastrointestinal (GI) tract that primarily affects premature infants. The incidence of NEC varies between 6% and 10% on average in VLBW (birthweight ≤1500 g) preterm infants admitted to neonatal

Funding Sources: NIH funding for Dr Ambalavanan; Dixon Fellowship and IKARIA funding for Dr Ramani.
There are no conflicts of interest.
a Department of Pediatrics, Women and Infants Center, University of Alabama at Birmingham, 176F Suite 9380, 619 South 19th Street, Birmingham, AL 35249-7335, USA; b Molecular and Cellular Pathology, University of Alabama at Birmingham, 176F Suite 9380, 619 South 19th Street, Birmingham, AL 35249–7335, USA; c Department of Cell, Developmental and Integrative Biology, University of Alabama at Birmingham, 176F Suite 9380, 619 South 19th Street, Birmingham, AL 35249–7335, USA
* Corresponding author. Department of Cell, Developmental, and Integrative Biology, Women and Infants Center, University of Alabama at Birmingham, 176F Suite 9380, 619 South 19th Street, Birmingham, AL 35249-7335.
E-mail address: ambal@uab.edu

intensive care units (NICUs) in the United States.[1-3] Despite remarkable advances in the care of extremely premature infants, the morbidity and mortality (10%–30%) caused by NEC has not declined significantly,[2,3] and the total cost of care is estimated to be as much as $1 billion annually in the United States alone.[3] NEC is a multifactorial disease in which the integrity and function of the immature GI tract are compromised as a result of prematurity, inflammation, ischemia, or abnormal gut microbiota (described in other articles elsewhere in this issue). Various feeding practices, such as the nature of feeds (human milk vs formula feeding), time of initiation of enteral feeds, and the rate at which at feeds are advanced, may also affect the immature GI tract and lead to the development of NEC.

Currently, there is no consensus among health care professionals on feeding practices in preterm infants and there are wide variations in such practices across NICUs in the United States. A recent survey of NICU directors, fellowship directors, neonatologists, neonatal nurse practitioners, and dieticians across NICUs in the United States indicated that most of responders would start parenteral nutrition on day 1 and the first enteral feed as soon as possible after birth (day 1: nonventilated; day 3: ventilated), either as human milk (56%) or commercially available formula.[4] Responders indicated they would consider indomethacin use (83%), history of *patent ductus arteriosus* (72%), and dopamine administration (63%) as contraindications for enteral feeding but not the placement of *umbilical artery catheter* (75%) or *umbilical venous catheter* (93%) or concurrent administration of hydrocortisone (70%).[4] Some of these feeding practices are not evidence based but based on personal experience or unit culture. The objective of this article is to review the current data on various feeding practices and their impact on risk of NEC, mortality, and other morbidities in preterm infants. This article identifies and examines several feeding practices that are proved safe or unsafe or remain unproved in the prevention of NEC. Recent randomized control trials, case-control studies, observational studies, and expert opinions on feeding practices and NEC in preterm infants are reviewed. For each subsection, quality of evidence is indicated (based on the US Preventive Services Task Force hierarchy of research design available at http://www.uspreventiveservicestaskforce.org/uspstf08/methods/procmanual4.htm) and a recommendation offered (based on the US Preventive Services Task Force definitions available at http://www.uspreventiveservicestaskforce.org/uspstf/grades.htm).

EFFECT OF HUMAN MILK VERSUS FORMULA FEEDING ON NEC

Preterm formulas that are available today have been designed to match the composition of human milk with respect to calories and nutrients that are needed for the growth and development of preterm infants. These synthesized formulas, however, do not provide the nonnutrient components of human milk, such as secretory IgA, lysozyme, oligosaccharides, polyunsaturated fatty acids, and platelet-activating factor acetylhydrolase. These non-nutrient components of human milk contribute to GI mucosal integrity and function and boost immunity against various GI infections. The American Academy of Pediatrics policy statement in 2012 on breastfeeding and the use of human milk recommends human milk for term, preterm, and other high-risk infants either by direct breastfeeding and or by expressed breast milk.[5] The American Academy of Pediatrics statement also indicated that donor human milk might be a suitable alternative for infants whose mothers are unable or unwilling to provide their own milk.[5]

There are many data suggesting that human milk provides long-term benefits in term infants by lowering the incidence of sudden infant death syndrome, childhood infectious diseases (respiratory tract infections, otitis media, and GI infection), allergic diseases, celiac disease, inflammatory bowel disease, obesity, and so forth.[5] In addition to these long-term benefits, preterm infants may benefit in the short term from the non-nutritive components of human milk by reduced susceptibility to sepsis or to NEC. There are currently no randomized controlled studies, however, comparing the effect of mother's own milk (not donor milk) with formula on the incidence of NEC and mortality.[6]

Several randomized controlled trials have been done to study the effect of donor human milk versus formula on the incidence of NEC and mortality in preterm infants. Meta-analysis of 5 of those randomized controlled trials comparing donor milk versus formula feeds in preterm infants showed that preterm infants fed with formula had more than twice the incidence of NEC (relative risk 2.5 [95% CI, 1.2–5.1] and number needed to harm 33 [95% CI, 17–100]) compared with the preterm infants fed with human milk.[7] The results of this meta-analysis underscore the importance of human milk intake in preterm infants.

Even though human milk intake reduces the risk of NEC, such reductions can only be achieved if preterm infants receive a certain minimal volume or proportion of their enteral feed as human milk. This dose-related benefit of human milk intake was evaluated in a secondary analysis of 1272 extremely low-birth-weight (ELBW) infants enrolled in the National Institute of Child Health and Human Development Glutamine Trial.[8] In this study population, approximately 13% of ELBW infants died or developed NEC 14 days after birth. For each 10% increase in the proportion of total intake as human milk, there was a reduction in NEC or death after 14 days by a factor of 0.83 (95% CI, 0.72–0.96).[8]

Similar results were also shown in a prospective cohort study by Sisk and colleagues,[9] in which 10% of VLBW infants who received less than 50% of their total enteral intake as human milk developed NEC whereas only 3% of infants who received more than 50% as human milk developed NEC. The odds of NEC decreased by 38% for every 25% increase in proportion of human milk in the first 14 days.[9] Overall, after adjustment for gestational age, higher human milk intake was associated with a lower risk of NEC (odds ratio 0.17 [95% CI, 0.04–0.68]; $P<.01$).[9]

Quality of evidence (I)

Recommendation grade (A)

The evidence is strong in favor of human milk (donor) compared with artificial formula in reducing the incidence of NEC in preterm infants. Even though such benefit is yet to be proved for a mother's own milk by randomized controlled trials, the authors can strongly recommend, based on existing evidence from donor human milk, that mothers should be encouraged and persuaded to feed preterm infants preferably with their own milk or with donor human milk if they are unable or unwilling to feed with their own milk.

EFFECT OF MINIMAL ENTERAL NUTRITION ON NEC

In utero, a fetus constantly swallows amniotic fluid, which contributes to the formation of meconium. In addition to the formation of meconium, amniotic fluid may also play an important role in growth and development of GI tract.[10] Postnatally, enteral feedings also stimulate the motility of the GI tract and various hormonal secretions.[11–13]

Fasting or delayed introduction of feeding may possibly impair these GI functions. To minimize feeding intolerance and the risk of developing NEC in preterm infants, the practice of MEN is considered as an alternative to complete fasting in many units.

MEN, otherwise called trophic feeds or gut priming, is usually started within 1 to 3 days after birth with 15 mL/kg/d to 20 mL/kg/d of enteral milk given every 2 to 3 hours and continued for 5 to 7 days after birth without any advancement. A recent Cochrane systematic review evaluated the effect of MEN on feeding intolerance, growth, incidence of NEC, and mortality in 754 VLBW infants.[14] Early trophic feeding was defined as enteral feeding with milk volume of up to 24 mL/kg/d began within 96 hours after birth and continued for at least 1 week whereas enteral fasting was defined as nothing per mouth for at least 1 week after birth. It was observed that there were no differences in the risk of developing NEC (relative risk [RR] 1.07 [95% CI, 0.67–1.7]; risk difference [RD] 0.01 [95% CI, 0.03–0.05]), time to achieve full feeds (weighted mean difference −0.97 [95% CI, −2.47 to −0.53]); mortality (RR 0.77 [95% CI, 0.46–1.30]; RD −0.03 [95% CI, 0.09–0.03]), and duration of hospital stay (weighted mean difference −3.8 days [95% CI, −12.2–4.5]) between VLBW infants who received minimal enteral feeding within 1 to 4 days after birth compared with complete enteral fasting for 7 days after birth.[14] Despite biologic plausibility that MEN may prime the gut and improve feeding intolerance and may thereby reduce the incidence of NEC, the data from available trials do not confirm that MEN in preterm infants improves feeding tolerance and reduces NEC.

Quality of evidence (I)

Recommendation grade (B)

The clinical importance of MEN is still uncertain, although it is commonly practiced. Based on the existing evidence that MEN (trophic feeds) does not increase the risk of NEC or feeding intolerance, MEN may be considered a safe alternative to complete fasting before the initiation of progressive feeding increments.

EFFECT OF RATE OF INCREMENT IN FEEDINGS ON NEC

NEC in preterm infants usually occurs a few weeks after birth.[2,3,15] At that time of diagnosis of NEC, most preterm infants have received enteral feeding, either with human milk or formula. Due to initial concerns that NEC may be associated with rapid advancement of enteral feeding,[16] many clinicians in the past have delayed initiating and slowed the rate of advancement of enteral feeding.

A Cochrane systematic review analyzed 5 randomized controlled trials involving 600 VLBW infants for the effect of delayed versus early progressive feeding on the incidence of NEC, mortality, and morbidities of preterm infants (growth, neurodevelopmental outcome, feeding intolerance, time to achieve full feeds, and length of hospital study).[17] "Delayed introduction of progressive feeds" was defined as intention to advance feed volumes in excess of trophic feeds (up to 24 mL/kg/d) later than 5 to 7 days after birth compared with advancing feeds at less than 4 days after birth. Two of the 5 randomized controlled trials (n = 488) recruited only growth-restricted infants with abnormal fetal circulatory distribution or flow in middle cerebral artery, umbilical arteries, or uterine arteries. Delayed advancement of enteral feedings in preterm infants did not have a significant effect on the risk of NEC (RR 0.89 [95% CI, 0.58–1.37) or all-cause mortality (RR 0.93 [95% CI, 0.53–1.63]).[17] In addition, preterm infants who received delayed advancement of feeds took longer to achieve full feeds (mean difference of 3 days) compared with those who have received feeds from earlier than four days after birth.[17] Data from these trials do not provide evidence that delayed introduction of progressive enteral feeds reduces the risk of NEC in VLBW infants and, moreover, results in several days delay in establishing full feeds. Rather than the exact rate of feed advancement, it is possible that the use of a standardized feeding regimen is more important. A systematic review of 6 observational studies by Patole and de Klerk[18] showed a reduction in the incidence of NEC by 87% (RR 0.13 [95% CI, 0.0–0.05]) with the use of a standardized feeding protocol.

Quality of evidence (I)

Recommendation grade (B)

Based on the existing evidence, early advancements of feeding is safe and may be considered an alternative to MEN soon after birth in clinically stable VLBW infants.

FEEDING ADVANCEMENT AND NEC

Enteral feeding is often advanced after 3 to 7 days of tolerance to MEN. The volume and the rate used to advance from MEN to full feeds vary between units and it usually depends on the birthweight and the extent of cardiorespiratory support. A daily increment between 15 mL/kg/d and 30 mL/kg/d of feeds is used in most units. A meta-analysis of 4 randomized controlled trials (n = 496; less than 1500 g or less than 32 weeks' gestational age) evaluated the effect of slow (15–20 mL/kg/d) versus fast (30–35 mL/kg/d) rates of enteral feed advancements on the incidence of NEC, mortality, and other morbidities in preterm infants.[19] No significant difference in the risk of NEC (RR 0.91 [95% CI, 0.47–1.75]; RD −0.01 [95% CI, −0.05–0.04]); and mortality (RR 1.43 [95% CI, 0.78–2.61]; RD 0.04 [95% CI, −0.02–0.09]) were noted between the slow and fast advancement groups.[19] Infants who were fed slowly took longer to regain birthweight (mean difference 2–6 days) and establish full feeds (2–5 days) compared with those who received more aggressive advancement of feeds. Data from this analysis do not provide evidence that slow advancement of feeds reduces NEC. In addition, slower advancement of feeds slows weight gain and establishment of full feeds. There may, therefore, be indirect effects on neonatal morbidity due to slow weight gain, delay in establishment of full feeds, prolongation of total parenteral nutrition, and risk of central line infection. These studies, however, did not include many severely growth-restricted infants or those with birthweight less than 750 g, and many clinicians increase feeds cautiously in this subgroup of infants.

Quality of evidence (I)

Recommendation grade (B)

Evidence indicates that both slow (15–20 mL/kg/d) and fast (30–35 mL/kg/d) advancement practices are safe and can be used in preterm infants (especially larger VLBW infants) while advancing MEN to full feeds. Randomized controlled trials are needed to determine the effect of slow versus fast feeding advancement on longer-term clinical outcomes of preterm infants and on the incidence of NEC and mortality in the subset of smaller ELBW infants (<750 g).

CONTINUOUS VERSUS INTERMITTENT BOLUS FEEDING ON NEC

Coordination of sucking and swallowing matures at approximately 32 to 34 weeks of gestation. Hence, tube feeding is usually necessary in VLBW infants to ensure adequate milk intake for growth and development. Tube feeding may be either intermittent (bolus) or continuous, with a set volume per hour. Intermittent enteral feeding may be more physiologic because it facilitates the normal cyclic surges of the GI hormones.[20,21] Continuous enteral feeding may, however, reduce the energy required for digestion and absorption and decrease feeding intolerance. The Cochrane systematic review, which included 7 trials that enrolled 511 VLBW infants and did not show any difference in the incidence of NEC (RR 1.5 [95% CI, 0.4–5.9]), time to achieve full enteral feeds (weighted mean difference 2 days [95% CI, −0.3–3.9]), and somatic growth between infants who were fed continuously and by intermittent tube feeding.[22] Available data do not provide evidence to determine best tube feeding practice in VLBW infants.

Quality of evidence (I)

Recommendation grade (B)

Even though intermittent feeding may have some physiologic advantages compared with continuous feeding, there is not enough evidence to recommend intermittent feeding versus continuous feeding for reducing the risk of NEC, mortality, or morbidity in preterm infants.

RELATIONSHIP OF FEEDING INTOLERANCE AND NEC

Feeding intolerance is common among preterm infants who are on enteral feeds and may either be a benign sign of reduced GI tract motility or an initial manifestation of NEC. Feeding intolerance is the one of most common reasons to delay advancement of enteral feeds or for suspension of feeds in preterm infants. There is no consensus, however, on the definition and management of feeding intolerance. Usually, an increased amount or abnormal nature (eg, bilious or bloody) of gastric residuals or abdominal distension regardless of gastric residuals is considered feeding intolerance. A case-control study by Cobb and colleagues[23] evaluating 51 infants with proved NEC versus 102 control infants without suspected or proved NEC indicated that a gastric residual volume of less than 1.5 mL or less than 25% of a feed (the 25th percentile for the NEC group) was probably within the range of normal but a gastric residual volume greater than 3.5 mL or greater than 33% of a feed (75th percentile for control subjects) was associated with a higher risk for NEC. There is no evidence that color (green vs milky) and or nature (mucus vs clear) of gastric residuals are early signs of NEC. Abdominal distension or visible loops may be a normal finding in preterm infants on continuous positive airway pressure and cannot be used as sole indicator in the diagnosis of NEC. Delayed advancement or suspension of enteral feeds based on gastric residuals or abdominal distension in the absence of other signs of NEC has not been shown to reduce the subsequent incidence of NEC. A retrospective chart analysis by Terrin and colleagues[24] to determine the safety and efficacy of MEN in feed-intolerant VLBW infants suggested that stopping or holding enteral feeds on the basis of feeding intolerance would increase the risk for sepsis (33.3% in the group restricted to nothing by mouth and 15.7% in MEN group; $P<.038$), days to achieve the full feeds (mean days = 11 in the group restricted to nothing by mouth and 8 in the MEN group; $P<.001$), and days to regain birthweight (mean days = 12 in the group restricted to nothing by mouth and 8 in the MEM group; $P<.001$).[24]

Quality of evidence (II-2)

Recommendation grade (I)

Currently, there is no evidence-based definition of feeding intolerance. A sudden increase in gastric residuals may be an early sign of NEC,[23] but abdominal distension and abnormal color or nature of gastric residuals are usually nonspecific. If clinically stable infants develop feeding intolerance in the absence of any other clinical or radiologic evidence of NEC, MEN (trophic feeds) may be provided while continuing to re-evaluate infants at frequent intervals, rather than suspending enteral feeding altogether.

EFFECT OF FORTIFIERS ON NEC

Preterm infants have higher protein turnover compared with term infants. Protein requirements for enterally fed preterm infants are inversely proportional to the body weight (ie, the lower the body weight, the higher the protein requirement).[25] Even at full feeds (200 mL/kg/d), the protein, calcium, and phosphorous content of human milk are not adequate to promote and sustain the tissue growth and bone mineraliza-tion in preterm infants.[26,27] Addition of fortifier increases levels of protein, calcium, and phosphorous of human milk. It has been shown that the multicomponent fortification of human milk is associated with short-term improvements in weight gain and linear and head growth.[28] There is a nonsignificant trend, however, toward increased feeding intolerance in treated infants (RR 2.85 [95% CI, 0.62–13.1]). There was no statistically significant increase in NEC in infants receiving fortified human milk (RR 1.33 [95% CI, 0.7–2.5]).[28]

Human milk can be fortified with either a human milk–based fortifier or bovine milk–based fortifier. To study the effect of exclusive human milk–based diet on the risk of NEC, Sullivan and colleagues[29] performed a randomized controlled trial involving 207 VLBW infants fed with either exclusive human milk–based diet or bovine-based diet. Exclusive human milk–based diet infants were fed only with either mother's own milk or human donor milk fortified only with donor human milk–based fortifier. Another group of infants were fed with mother's own milk or human donor milk fortified with bovine-based human milk fortifier. A third group (control) received mother's own milk fortified with bovine-based human milk fortifier and received preterm formula when mother's own milk was not available. The group receiving exclusive human milk diet had lower rates of NEC ($P = .02$) and NEC requiring surgical intervention ($P = .007$) compared with the group receiving human milk fortified with bovine-based fortifier.[29] Limitations of this study, however, were small sample size and higher incidence of NEC in the control group (18%).[2,3]

Quality of evidence (I)

Recommendation grade (B)

Currently, limited evidence suggests that fortification of human milk improves short-term growth moderately without a significant increase in NEC or improved long-term outcomes. There is also some evidence that human milk–based fortifier reduces the incidence of NEC. The high cost and unknown biologic product risks associated with human milk–based fortifier currently limit its routine use in fortifying human milk.

EFFECT OF OSMOLALITY OF FEEDS ON NEC

Osmolality is the concentration of a solution in terms of osmoles of solute per kilogram of solvent, whereas osmolarity is the concentration of a solution in terms of osmoles of solute per liter of solution. Current recommendations mostly based on historical consensus rather than experimental evidence are that the osmolality of enteral feeds should not exceed 450 mOsm/kg (approximately 400 mOsm/L).[30,31] The recommen-dations seem to have been mostly based on small studies in the 1970s by Santulli and colleagues,[32] Book and colleagues,[33] and Willis and colleagues.[34] Human breast milk has an osmolality of approximately 300 mOsm/kg, whereas that of full-fortified human milk is approximately 400 mOsm/kg, and all milk feeds that are currently used have an osmolality below 450 mOsm/kg.[30] The addition of supplements (eg, sodium supple-ments and folate), however, may markedly increase osmolality, with the exact magni-tude depending on the amount of supplement and the volume of milk to which it is added.[35] The consequences of increased feed osmolality in human infants are not clear. Studies in neonatal dogs indicate that the actual osmolality of the feed itself was not a major determinant of the osmolality of the contents of the stomach or intes-tine, although hyperosmolar feeds led to delayed gastric emptying.[36] Even if hyperos-molar feeds led to increased hyperosmolarity in the intestinal lumen, it is not clear that this would result in mucosal damage.[30]

Quality of evidence (II-3)

Recommendation grade (B)

Studies that showed the association of increased incidence of NEC with hyperosmolar formula feedings were done at a time when osmolality of the feeds were high and above the current recommended maximum (450 mOsm/kg). The increase in osmolality of enteral feedings by the addition of supplements and other therapeutic additives may possibly result in delayed gastric emptying, with an undetermined effect on NEC.

SUMMARY

The evidence is convincing that human milk feeding, compared with formula feeding, reduces the incidence of NEC in preterm infants. MEN is a safe alternative to complete fasting before initiation of progressive feedings and does not increase the incidence of NEC in extremely preterm infants. In clinically stable VLBW infants, early introduction of progressive feeds and advancement of feeds at a faster rate (30–35 mL/kg/d) is safe and does not increase the incidence of NEC. There is no evidence supporting continuous versus intermittent tube feedings in preterm infants. In feed-intolerant preterm infants without any other clinical and radiologic evidence of NEC, MEN rather than complete suspension of enteral feeding may be an alternative. Human milk–based fortifier compared with bovine-based fortifier may reduce the incidence of NEC but additional studies are required.

REFERENCES

1. Guillet R, Stoll BJ, Cotten CM, et al. Association of H2-blocker therapy and higher incidence of necrotizing enterocolitis in very low birth weight infants. Pediatrics 2006;117(2):e137–42.
2. Lin PW, Stoll BJ. Necrotising enterocolitis. Lancet 2006;368(9543):1271–83.
3. Neu J, Walker WA. Necrotizing enterocolitis. N Engl J Med 2011;364(3): 255–64.
4. Hans DM, Pylipow M, Long JD, et al. Nutritional practices in the neonatal intensive care unit: analysis of a 2006 neonatal nutrition survey. Pediatrics 2009; 123(1):51–7.
5. Section on Breastfeeding. Breastfeeding and the use of human milk. Pediatrics 2012;129(3):e827–41.
6. Henderson G, Anthony MY, McGuire W. Formula milk versus maternal breast milk for feeding preterm or low birth weight infants. Cochrane Database Syst Rev 2007;(4):CD002972.
7. Quigley MA, Henderson G, Anthony MY, et al. Formula milk versus donor breast milk for feeding preterm or low birth weight infants. Cochrane Database Syst Rev 2007;(4):CD002971.
8. Meinzen-Derr J, Poindexter B, Wrage L, et al. Role of human milk in extremely low birth weight infants' risk of necrotizing enterocolitis or death. J Perinatol 2009; 29(1):57–62.
9. Sisk PM, Lovelady CA, Dillard RG, et al. Early human milk feeding is associated with a lower risk of necrotizing enterocolitis in very low birth weight infants. J Perinatol 2007;27(7):428–33.
10. Trahair JF, Harding R. Ultrastructural anomalies in the fetal small intestine indicate that fetal swallowing is important for normal development: an experimental study. Virchows Arch A Pathol Anat Histopathol 1992;420(4):305–12.

11. Johnson LR. The trophic action of gastrointestinal hormones. Gastroenterology 1976;70(2):278–88.
12. Lucas A, Bloom SR, Aynsley-Green A. Gut hormones and 'minimal enteral feeding'. Acta Paediatr Scand 1986;75(5):719–23.
13. Berseth CL. Neonatal small intestinal motility: motor responses to feeding in term and preterm infants. J Pediatr 1990;117(5):777–82.
14. Bombell S, McGuire W. Early trophic feeding for very low birth weight infants. Cochrane Database Syst Rev 2009;(3):CD000504.
15. Uauy RD, Fanaroff AA, Korones SB, et al. Necrotizing enterocolitis in very low birth weight infants: biodemographic and clinical correlates. National Institute of Child Health and Human Development Neonatal Research Network. J Pediatr 1991;119(4):630–8.
16. Anderson DM, Kliegman RM. The relationship of neonatal alimentation practices to the occurrence of endemic necrotizing enterocolitis. Am J Perinatol 1991;8(1): 62–7.
17. Morgan J, Young L, McGuire W. Delayed introduction of progressive enteral feeds to prevent necrotising enterocolitis in very low birth weight infants. Cochrane Database Syst Rev 2011;(3):CD001970.
18. Patole SK, de Klerk N. Impact of standardised feeding regimens on incidence of neonatal necrotising enterocolitis: a systematic review and meta-analysis of observational studies. Arch Dis Child Fetal Neonatal Ed 2005;90(2):F147–51.
19. Morgan J, Young L, McGuire W. Slow advancement of enteral feed volumes to prevent necrotising enterocolitis in very low birth weight infants. Cochrane Database Syst Rev 2011;(3):CD001241.
20. Strader AD, Woods SC. Gastrointestinal hormones and food intake. Gastroenterology 2005;128(1):175–91.
21. Aynsley-Green A, Adrian TE, Bloom SR. Feeding and the development of enteroinsular hormone secretion in the preterm infant: effects of continuous gastric infusions of human milk compared with intermittent boluses. Acta Paediatr Scand 1982;71(3):379–83.
22. Premji SS, Chessell L. Continuous nasogastric milk feeding versus intermittent bolus milk feeding for premature infants less than 1500 grams. Cochrane Database Syst Rev 2011;(11):CD001819.
23. Cobb BA, Carlo WA, Ambalavanan N. Gastric residuals and their relationship to necrotizing enterocolitis in very low birth weight infants. Pediatrics 2004; 113(1 Pt 1):50–3.
24. Terrin G, Passariello A, Canani RB, et al. Minimal enteral feeding reduces the risk of sepsis in feed-intolerant very low birth weight newborns. Acta Paediatr 2009; 98(1):31–5.
25. Ziegler EE. Protein requirements of very low birth weight infants. J Pediatr Gastroenterol Nutr 2007;45(Suppl 3):S170–4.
26. Cohen RS, McCallie KR. Feeding premature infants: why, when, and what to add to human milk. JPEN J Parenter Enteral Nutr 2012;36(Suppl 1):20S–4S.
27. Schanler RJ. Evaluation of the evidence to support current recommendations to meet the needs of premature infants: the role of human milk. Am J Clin Nutr 2007; 85(2):625S–8S.
28. Kuschel CA, Harding JE. Multicomponent fortified human milk for promoting growth in preterm infants. Cochrane Database Syst Rev 2004;(1):CD000343.
29. Sullivan S, Schanler RJ, Kim JH, et al. An exclusively human milk-based diet is associated with a lower rate of necrotizing enterocolitis than a diet of human milk and bovine milk-based products. J Pediatr 2010;156(4):562–567.e1.

30. Pearson F, Johnson MJ, Leaf AA. Milk osmolality: does it matter? Arch Dis Child Fetal Neonatal Ed 2011. [Epub ahead of print].
31. Commentary on breast-feeding and infant formulas, including proposed standards for formulas. Pediatrics 1976;57(2):278–85.
32. Santulli TV, Schullinger JN, Heird WC, et al. Acute necrotizing enterocolitis in infancy: a review of 64 cases. Pediatrics 1975;55(3):376–87.
33. Book LS, Herbst JJ, Atherton SO, et al. Necrotizing enterocolitis in low-birth-weight infants fed an elemental formula. J Pediatr 1975;87(4):602–5.
34. Willis DM, Chabot J, Radde IC, et al. Unsuspected hyperosmolality of oral solutions contributing to necrotizing enterocolitis in very-low-birth-weight infants. Pediatrics 1977;60(4):535–8.
35. Srinivasan L, Bokiniec R, King C, et al. Increased osmolality of breast milk with therapeutic additives. Arch Dis Child Fetal Neonatal Ed 2004;89(6):F514–7.
36. Goldblum OM, Holzman IR, Fisher SE. Intragastric feeding in the neonatal dog. Its effect on intestinal osmolality. Am J Dis Child 1981;135(7):631–3.

Therapeutic Use of Prebiotics, Probiotics, and Postbiotics to Prevent Necrotizing Enterocolitis
What is the Current Evidence?

Ravi Mangal Patel, MD, Patricia Wei Denning, MD*

KEYWORDS

- Necrotizing enterocolitis • Probiotic bacteria • Premature infants
- Very low birth weight

KEY POINTS

- Current evidence suggests that probiotics are effective in decreasing NEC in preterm infants.
- Concerns regarding safety and optimal dosing have limited the routine clinical use of probiotics in preterm infants.
- Prebiotics and postbiotics are potential alternatives or adjunctive therapies to the administration of live microorganisms, although studies demonstrating their clinical efficacy in preventing NEC are currently lacking.

INTRODUCTION: NECROTIZING ENTEROCOLITIS

Necrotizing enterocolitis (NEC) is a leading cause of neonatal morbidity and mortality, and the most common gastrointestinal emergency in neonates.[1,2] NEC develops in approximately 1 of 10 infants born at less than 29 weeks' gestation.[3] Approximately 20% to 30% of very low birth weight (≤1500 g) infants who develop NEC die,[4] and those infants who survive the disease are at risk for long-term complications, including neurodevelopmental impairment, short bowel syndrome, and impaired growth.[5] Considerable health costs result, with the financial impact of affected infants in the

Disclosures: The authors do not have any relevant disclosures.
Grant support: Supported by the National Center for Advancing Translational Sciences of the National Institutes of Health (NIH) under Award Number UL1TR000454 (R.M.P.) and NIH R01 HD059122 (P.W.D). The content is solely the responsibility of the authors and does not necessarily represent the official views of the National Institutes of Health.
Division of Neonatal-Perinatal Medicine, Department of Pediatrics, Emory University School of Medicine, 2015 Uppergate Drive Northeast, 3rd Floor, Atlanta, GA 30322, USA
* Corresponding author.
E-mail address: pllin@emory.edu

United States estimated to be between \$500 million and \$1 billion per year.[6] NEC is particularly poignant for families because it affects preterm infants who have survived the initial postnatal period only to develop a new and life-threatening illness.

NEC is characterized by intestinal injury, inflammation, and necrosis. Despite investigative efforts, the underlying pathogenesis remains unclear. Leading hypotheses implicate a multifactorial pathophysiology, which includes host factors, inflammatory propensity of the immature gut, enteral feeding, and abnormal bacterial colonization (**Box 1**).[6-8] NEC can rapidly progress from early clinical signs to extensive intestinal necrosis within hours, limiting the effectiveness of therapeutic intervention. As such, approaches to prevent NEC have become a focus of research efforts, and preventive therapies for NEC are urgently needed.[9]

Probiotics are the most promising treatment on the horizon for this devastating disease. However, further study is needed, as reviewed in this article, before probiotics can be routinely recommended as a preventive therapy. In addition, prebiotics and postbiotics remain potential alternatives or adjunctive therapies to the use of live microorganisms. This article reviews the role of microorganisms in intestinal heath and disease in neonates, and the current evidence supporting prebiotic, probiotic, and postbiotic use in preterm infants. In addition, the potential mechanisms of action of probiotic organisms are discussed and the risks and benefits of therapy are weighed. Important terminology is defined in **Box 2**.

ROLE OF INTESTINAL MICROORGANISMS IN INTESTINAL DEVELOPMENT AND HEALTH

The neonatal intestine is the largest interface of the host to the external environment. Ideally the intestine protects the vulnerable neonate from pathogens and toxins while allowing harmonious habitation of commensal bacteria. In addition, the intestine must protect itself from bacterial pathogens that cause inflammation while encouraging the growth and habitation of commensal bacteria, which can attenuate inflammation and maintain intestinal homeostasis.[10] Of importance, uncontrolled inflammation can lead to tissue injury and necrosis, and is thought to play an important role in the pathogenesis of NEC.[6]

The immature neonatal gut in the preterm infant has even greater challenges as it transitions from a sterile lumen absent of microbes to the fully realized "bioreactor"

Box 1
Risk factors influencing NEC predisposition

- Prematurity
  - Inflammatory propensity of the immature gut[74-76]
  - Decreased intestinal barrier function[77,78]
  - Decreased gut motility and aberrant vascular regulation[79,80]
- Enteral feeding
  - Aggressive advancement of feeding[81,82]
  - Nonhuman milk feeding[83,84]
- Abnormal bacterial colonization
  - Prolonged empiric initial antibiotic therapy[21,23,24]
  - Decreased commensal flora[20,85]
  - Increased pathogenic bacteria[19,85]

Box 2
Key definitions

- *Probiotics* are supplements or foods that contain viable microorganisms that alter the microflora of the host.
- *Prebiotics* are supplements or foods that contain a nondigestible ingredient that selectively stimulates the growth and/or activity of indigenous bacteria.
- *Postbiotics* are nonviable bacterial products or metabolic byproducts from probiotic microorganisms that have biological activity in the host.
- *Synbiotic* is a product that contains both probiotics and prebiotics.

of the mature adult gut. Very soon after birth, a newborn infant's intestine begins to acquire a diverse set of commensal bacteria. These bacteria eventually grow to outnumber their host by a factor of 10 to 1.[11–13] The infant/host provides a hospitable, temperature-stable, nutrient-rich environment for bacteria while receiving, in return, benefits from the commensal bacteria, which include digestion, absorption, and storage of nutrients,[14,15] intestinal homeostasis and protection against injury,[13,16] and the development and control of epithelial immune responses and function.[17,18] However, this postnatal transition from a sterile to commensal-rich intestine may become disrupted or delayed in infants born prematurely.

ABNORMAL BACTERIAL COLONIZATION IN PRETERM INFANTS

Premature infants, when compared with their term counterparts, are more likely to be colonized with fewer, more virulent organisms.[19] In addition, they have delayed acquisition of commensal bacteria, particularly *Bifidobacteria*.[20] Several explanations are likely as to why this occurs (**Fig. 1**). Preterm infants and their mothers are commonly exposed to antibiotic therapy, both of which have been associated with an increased risk of NEC.[21–24] In addition, because preterm infants are often delivered by cesarean section and experience delayed enteral feeding, they are less likely to acquire commensal flora perinatally from passage through the birth canal or from human milk feeding; this may lead to decreased colonization of beneficial probiotic bacteria, including *Bifidobacteria*, *Lactobacillus*, and *Bacteroides*.[25,26] The hospital environment, with its preponderance of pathogenic organisms,[27] may also negatively affect the intestinal colonization of beneficial commensal bacteria. Ongoing studies investigating the intestinal microbiome in premature neonates will provide greater insight into

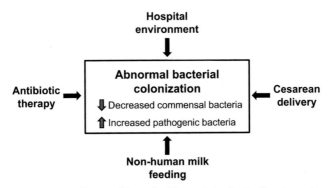

Fig. 1. Factors influencing abnormal intestinal bacterial colonization in preterm infants.

the role of microbial diversity on the development of NEC.[28–30] Because abnormal bacterial colonization likely plays a role in the pathogenesis of NEC, probiotic bacteria may exert their beneficial effects by restoring or supplying the essential commensal strains necessary for protection against intestinal inflammation and injury. Prebiotics and postbiotics may also accomplish this goal, through the promotion of commensal growth or by mirroring commensal activity, respectively.

MECHANISMS OF ACTION
Probiotics

In preterm infants, probiotic supplementation can allow acquisition of normal commensal flora in a host where this process has been delayed or support the transition to an intestinal microbiome with beneficial microbes, particularly in hosts where this process has been disrupted. Several mechanisms of probiotic action may explain how their therapeutic use can help prevent NEC. These mechanisms include enhancement of epithelial barrier function, competitive exclusion of pathogens, and direct anti-inflammatory effects on epithelial signaling pathways.[31–33] At the cellular level, probiotics have several important effects (**Fig. 2**): (1) attenuation of nuclear factor κB activation, a major proinflammatory pathway[34]; (2) upregulation of cytoprotective genes[13,35]; (3) prevention of apoptosis and cell death[35,36]; (4) generation of reactive oxygen species important in cell signaling[37,38]; and (5) induction of the expression of tight junction proteins necessary for barrier function.[39,40] Whether live microorganisms, instead of killed or inactivated bacteria or bacterial products, are required for these beneficial effects remains an important area of study, and recent data suggest that bacterial products, in the absence of viable organisms, may have similar effects on signaling pathways[41] and barrier function.[39] These bacterial products, broadly characterized as postbiotics, are discussed in a separate section.

Because the preterm gut demonstrates delayed commensal colonization and low bacterial diversity, it may be particularly amenable to therapeutic manipulation by probiotic administration. In keeping with this idea, several clinical studies have demonstrated the benefit of probiotic administration in reducing the incidence and severity of NEC (**Table 1**). Most of these trials have used strains of probiotics from the genus *Lactobacillus* or *Bifidobacteria,* although the treatment regimen, including dose and duration of therapy, vary widely (**Table 2**). In addition, concerns regarding the risks of therapy, optimal species or combination of species, duration of therapy, and dosing remain unanswered. The therapeutic use of probiotics is discussed later.

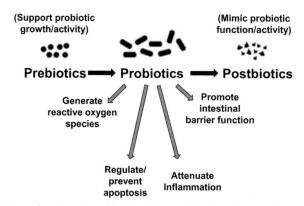

Fig. 2. Mechanisms of action of probiotics at the cellular level in intestinal epithelia.

Table 1
Summary of probiotic therapy trials in preterm infants

Study Authors,[Ref.] Year	No. of Infants	BW and/or GA	Primary Outcome of NEC
Kitajima et al,[86] 1997	91	<1500 g	No
Dani et al,[87] 2002	585	<1500 g or <33 wk	Yes
Costalos et al,[88] 2003	87	28–32 wk	No
Bin-Nun et al,[89] 2005	145	<1500 g	Yes
Lin et al,[90] 2005	367	<1500 g	Yes
Manzoni et al,[91] 2006	80	<1500 g	No
Mohan et al,[92] 2006	38 of 69[a]	<37 wk	No
Stratiki et al,[93] 2007	41 of 75[a]	27–36 wk	No
Lin et al,[69] 2008	434	<1500 g and <34 wk	Yes
Samanta et al,[68] 2009	186	<1500 g and <32 wk	Yes
Rouge et al,[94] 2009	94	<1500 g and <32 wk	No
Manzoni et al,[67] 2009	319 of 472	<1500 g	No
Underwood et al,[48] 2009	90	750–2000 g and <35 wk	No
Mihatsch et al,[95] 2010	183	<1500 g and <30 wk	No
Braga et al,[96] 2011	231	750–1499 g	Yes
Sari et al,[97] 2011	221	<1500 g or <33 wk	Yes
Fernandez-Carrocera et al,[98] 2012	150	<1500 g	Yes

Abbreviations: BW, birth weight; GA, gestational age; NEC, necrotizing enterocolitis.
[a] Only infants <34 wk and <1500 g included.
Data from individual studies referenced and from Deshpande G, Rao S, Patole S, et al. Updated meta-analysis of probiotics for preventing necrotizing enterocolitis in preterm neonates. Pediatrics 2010;125:921–30.

Prebiotics

Another potential therapeutic strategy to prevent NEC that may carry less infectious risk is prebiotic therapy. Prebiotics are nondigestible dietary products, which improve intestinal health by promoting selective growth of beneficial commensal bacteria.[42] The most common prebiotics are oligosaccharides, which are found in human milk. Prebiotics have been added to infant formulas in Japan for more than 2 decades, and there is increasing use of prebiotics in the commercial formula market in the United States, although concerns regarding their efficacy remain.[43,44] Several studies have demonstrated increased *Bifidobacteria* and decreased pathogenic bacteria in the stool of preterm infants fed prebiotic-containing formula with short-chain gal-acto-oligosaccharides (GOS) and/or fructo-oligosaccharides (FOS) in comparison with control infants.[45–47] Similar effects of increased *Bifidobacteria* colonization were seen with the use of synbiotics, which combine prebiotics with probiotics.[48] In addition to promoting the growth of beneficial commensals, prebiotic therapy may also improve intestinal motility and gastric emptying, resulting in improved feeding tolerance.[49,50] Evidence suggests that this effect of prebiotics on gastrointestinal motility is mediated by bacterial metabolites such as short-chain fatty acids[51] and, therefore, may actually be a postbiotic effect rather than a direct effect of the prebiotic. Term infants exhibit decreased stool pH and increased stool short-chain fatty acids when fed prebiotic-containing formula, reportedly comparable with that seen in breastfed infants.[52] In addition, preliminary evidence suggests a positive effect on

Table 2
Summary of probiotic strains used in therapeutic trials in preterm infants

Probiotic Genus	Species	Dose (CFU/day)	Reference
Bifidobacterium	bifidus	1×10^9 [a]	48,89
		2×10^9 [a]	69
		5×10^9 [a]	68
	breve	0.5×10^9	86
		3.5×10^7–3.5×10^9 [a]	96
	infantis	2.76×10^7 [a]	98
		1×10^9 [a]	48,89
		5×10^9 [a]	68
		NR	90
	lactis	2×10^7 [b]	93
		1.6–4.8×10^9	92
		1.2×10^{10}	95
	longus	4×10^8 [a]	94
		1×10^9 [a]	48
		5×10^9 [a]	68
Lactobacillus	acidophilus	1×10^9 [a]	48,98
		2×10^9 [a]	69
		5×10^9 [a]	68
		NR	90
	casei	1×10^9 [a]	98
		3.5×10^7–3.5×10^9 [a]	96
	rhamnosus GG	4×10^8	94
		4.4×10^8 [a]	98
		1×10^9	48
		6×10^9	67,87,91
	plantarum	1.76×10^8 [a]	98
	sporogenes	3.5×10^8	97
Streptococcus	theromphilus	6.6×10^5 [a]	98
		1×10^9 [a]	89
Saccharomyces	boulardii	2×10^9 per kg	88

Abbreviations: CFU, colony forming units; NR, not reported in CFU per day.
 [a] Indicates therapeutic use in combination with other probiotic species.
 [b] Dose is per gram of milk powder of preterm formula.

overall immune function.[53] Although no serious adverse effects of prebiotic therapy were noted in the previously mentioned studies, prebiotic therapy is associated with several gastrointestinal side effects including flatulence, bloating, and diarrhea, which can be reversed by stopping treatment.[42]

Postbiotics

Using bacterial products or metabolites remains an exciting, yet largely unexplored, therapeutic option for preventing NEC. Postbiotics aim to mimic the beneficial therapeutic effects of probiotics while avoiding the risk of administering live microorganisms to preterm infants with immature intestinal barriers or impaired immune defenses. Many commensal bacteria produce butyrate, a short-chain fatty acid produced by the catabolism of undigested carbohydrates in the intestine. Butyrate is a major energy source for the colon, and has an important role in intestinal growth and differentiation,[54,55] inflammatory suppression[56–58] (including suppression through generation of reactive oxygen species),[59] and regulation of apoptosis.[60,61] It has been used with limited success in inflammatory bowel disease.[62] Perhaps this and other small-molecule products of the normal flora are at least partially responsible for the beneficial effects of the normal flora (and exogenous probiotics and prebiotics), and could be used as a more controllable and safer therapeutic surrogate. Heat-killed probiotics may also function, in the broad sense, as postbiotics. Heat-killed microorganisms retain important bacterial structures that may exert biological activity in the host. The authors recently reported that heat-killed *Lactobacillus rhamnosus* GG (*LGG*) has beneficial efficacy similar to that of live probiotics in accelerating intestinal barrier maturation in a murine model of immature intestines.[39] More importantly, whereas administration of higher doses of live *LGG* led to increased mortality in immature neonatal mice, administration of heat-killed *LGG* did not.

THERAPEUTIC OPTIONS

Numerous probiotic organisms have been studied in preterm infants, at varied dosages and durations of therapy (see **Table 2**). The diversity of use has made the selection of an optimal probiotic regimen difficult. Several studies have used single agents, whereas several larger trials have used a combination of probiotics. Dosing varies among probiotic species and ranges from 10^5 to 10^{10} colony-forming units (CFU) per day. In addition, the actual probiotic composition may vary from what is advertised.[48] Most studies randomized infants and/or initiated therapy within a week after birth, and duration of therapy typically lasted beyond 1 month of age with several studies continuing therapy until hospital discharge. The 2 most commonly used probiotic strains were from the genera *Bifidobacteria* and *Lactobacillus*. A meta-analysis by Wang and colleagues,[63] including several recent trials conducted in China, compared the relative efficacy of these strains by pooling studies that used these probiotic agents, and found that *Bifidobacteria, Lactobacillus*, and a combination of the 2 strains had similar efficacy in the prevention of NEC (**Table 3**). Of note, monitoring for adverse effects varied greatly among the studies, particularly in those where NEC was not a primary outcome measure.

For prebiotics, several oligosaccharides including fructose, galactose, lactulose, inulin, or a combination of these are potential therapeutic options for clinical use.[64] GOS, FOS, and a combination of the two (GOS-FOS) have been used clinically in

Table 3			
Comparison of the efficacy of probiotic strains			
Outcome	Probiotic	Total Patients (N)	Pooled Relative Risk (95% CI)
NEC	*Lactobacillus*	1205	0.37 (0.19–0.73)
	Bifidobacteria	976	0.30 (0.16–0.58)
	Both	1403	0.33 (0.19–0.58)
Death	*Lactobacillus*	1205	0.61 (0.38–0.97)
	Bifidobacteria	340	0.74 (0.18–2.97)
	Both	1312	0.47 (0.26–0.87)
Sepsis	*Lactobacillus*	1205	0.79 (0.46–1.36)
	Bifidobacteria	340	0.84 (0.29–2.41)
	Both	1312	0.90 (0.60–1.36)

Abbreviations: CI, confidence interval; NEC, necrotizing enterocolitis.

Data from Wang Q, Dong J, Zhu Y. Probiotic supplement reduces risk of necrotizing enterocolitis and mortality in preterm very-low-birth-weight infants: an updated meta-analysis of 20 randomized, controlled trials. J Pediatr Surg 2012;47:241–8.

preterm infants, and studies have shown increased *Bifidobacteria* stool colony counts in prebiotic-treated infants, although none of these studies evaluated NEC as a primary outcome measure.[65]

CLINICAL OUTCOMES

Clinical trials have consistently demonstrated trends in favor of probiotic treatment, compared with placebo, in reducing the incidence of NEC (**Fig. 3**A). Four of these studies demonstrated a statistically significant benefit, and 2 recent meta-analyses of therapeutic trials have both shown similar pooled relative risks in favor of probiotics for the prevention of NEC. Deshpande and colleagues[66] evaluated 11 trials and found an overall pooled relative risk (RR) of 0.35 (95% confidence interval [CI] 0.23–0.55) for NEC in infants randomized to probiotic therapy compared with controls. Wang and

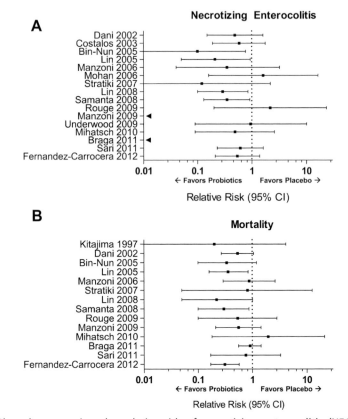

Fig. 3. Plots demonstrating the relative risk of necrotizing enterocolitis (NEC) (*A*) and mortality (*B*) in the probiotic treatment arm, compared with placebo, of therapeutic trials in preterm infants. Error bars reflect 95% confidence interval (CI) for relative risk estimates. Two studies had no NEC events in the probiotic treatment arm and estimates, without 95% CI, are indicated by black arrows. (*Data from* individual studies referenced as well as from Deshpande G, Rao S, Patole S, et al. Updated meta-analysis of probiotics for preventing necrotizing enterocolitis in preterm neonates. Pediatrics 2010;125:921–30; and Wang Q, Dong J, Zhu Y. Probiotic supplement reduces risk of necrotizing enterocolitis and mortality in preterm very-low-birth-weight infants: an updated meta-analysis of 20 randomized, controlled trials. J Pediatr Surg 2012;47:241–8.)

colleagues,[63] as mentioned previously, included more recent trials, and found a similar pooled RR of 0.33 (95% CI 0.24–0.46) from a total of 20 studies. Of note, only 8 of 17 trials identified had NEC listed as a primary outcome measure, and the dose and species of probiotics used varied widely (see **Tables 1** and **2**). Of importance, the previously mentioned meta-analyses also demonstrated a decreased risk of death (**Fig. 3**B) in infants randomized to probiotic treatment compared with control. It is likely that the mortality benefit is through a reduction in NEC-related and sepsis-related deaths, although the causes of death have not been routinely evaluated in clinical trials.

However, the benefit of probiotics in the prevention of sepsis (**Fig. 4**) is not as clear. Two randomized trials, including a large trial by Manzoni and colleagues,[67] have shown a benefit of probiotics in reducing late-onset sepsis.[68] However, Manzoni and colleagues[67] used the probiotic *LGG* in combination with lactoferrin and did not evaluate probiotic treatment alone. Other studies have shown no benefit, and one study showed an increased risk of sepsis with an RR of 1.67 (95% CI 1.04–2.67), raising concerns regarding the risk of sepsis with probiotic therapy.[69]

Although prebiotics and postbiotics are potential alternatives or supplements to probiotic therapy, no clinical trials have studied the therapeutic use of these substances for the prevention of NEC. Therefore, one can only speculate on the potential benefit of prebiotics and postbiotics in the preterm infant until more definitive data are available regarding their effects on important clinical outcomes of prematurity, such as NEC, sepsis, or death.

COMPLICATIONS AND CONCERNS

Although the clinical efficacy of probiotics in preventing NEC is promising, concerns regarding the complications associated with therapy have mitigated their widespread use. Probiotic use in premature infants could expose intestinal epithelia with poor defenses and a tendency toward inflammation to a microbial challenge too soon, resulting in inflammation, injury, or sepsis. Several reports of probiotic-associated

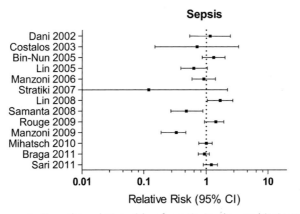

Fig. 4. Plot demonstrating the relative risk of sepsis in the probiotic treatment arm, compared with placebo, of therapeutic trials in preterm infants. Error bars reflect 95% confidence interval (CI) for relative risk estimates. (*Data from* individual studies referenced as well as from Deshpande G, Rao S, Patole S, et al. Updated meta-analysis of probiotics for preventing necrotizing enterocolitis in preterm neonates. Pediatrics 2010;125:921–30; and Wang Q, Dong J, Zhu Y. Probiotic supplement reduces risk of necrotizing enterocolitis and mortality in preterm very-low-birth-weight infants: an updated meta-analysis of 20 randomized, controlled trials. J Pediatr Surg 2012;47:241–8.)

sepsis[70–72] have raised concerns regarding routine clinical use of live bacteria in hosts, such as premature infants, who have immature epithelial-barrier defenses. The American Academy of Pediatrics Committee on Nutrition—Section on Gastroenterology, Hepatology, and Nutrition[73] and the ESPGHAN Committee on Nutrition[44] both have highlighted the need for large, well-designed clinical research studies before widespread use is adopted. The use of prebiotics or postbiotics may decrease these concerns regarding safety. However, no data from trials of prebiotics or postbiotics for the prevention of NEC in preterm infants are currently available. In addition, these agents are likely to encounter issues regarding optimal dosing similar to those seen with probiotic therapy.

SUMMARY

NEC remains a devastating complication of prematurity, and new preventive therapies are urgently needed. Probiotic therapy has demonstrated promising efficacy for the prevention of NEC, as evidenced by a very strong treatment effect in favor of probiotic therapy in 2 recent meta-analyses.[63,66] However, safety and dosing concerns continue to temper widespread use, and these concerns are likely to remain until large, multicenter trials adequately designed to address safety are completed. In addition, the use of prebiotics or postbiotics may be potential alternatives to the use of live probiotic organisms, although the therapeutic benefit of these products in preventing NEC remains largely unknown. Further studies are needed to guide clinicians on the use of probiotics, prebiotics, and postbiotics for the prevention of NEC.

REFERENCES

1. Henry MC, Moss LR. Necrotizing enterocolitis. Annu Rev Med 2009;60:111–24.
2. Lin PW, Stoll BJ. Necrotising enterocolitis. Lancet 2006;368:1271–83.
3. Stoll BJ, Hansen NI, Bell EF, et al. Neonatal outcomes of extremely preterm infants from the NICHD Neonatal Research Network. Pediatrics 2010;126:443–56.
4. Fitzgibbons SC, Ching Y, Yu D, et al. Mortality of necrotizing enterocolitis expressed by birth weight categories. J Pediatr Surg 2009;44:1072–5 [discussion: 5–6].
5. Hintz SR, Kendrick DE, Stoll BJ, et al. Neurodevelopmental and growth outcomes of extremely low birth weight infants after necrotizing enterocolitis. Pediatrics 2005;115:696–703.
6. Neu J, Walker WA. Necrotizing enterocolitis. N Engl J Med 2011;364:255–64.
7. Lin PW, Nasr TR, Stoll BJ. Necrotizing enterocolitis: recent scientific advances in pathophysiology and prevention. Semin Perinatol 2008;32:70–82.
8. Patel RM, Lin PW. Developmental biology of gut-probiotic interaction. Gut Microbes 2010;1:186–95.
9. Grave GD, Nelson SA, Walker WA, et al. New therapies and preventive approaches for necrotizing enterocolitis: report of a research planning workshop. Pediatr Res 2007;62:510–4.
10. Collier-Hyams LS, Neish AS. Innate immune relationship between commensal flora and the mammalian intestinal epithelium. Cell Mol Life Sci 2005;62:1339–48.
11. Backhed F, Ley RE, Sonnenburg JL, et al. Host-bacterial mutualism in the human intestine. Science 2005;307:1915–20.
12. Hooper LV, Gordon JI. Commensal host-bacterial relationships in the gut. Science 2001;292:1115–8.
13. Hooper LV, Wong MH, Thelin A, et al. Molecular analysis of commensal host-microbial relationships in the intestine. Science 2001;291:881–4.

14. Backhed F, Ding H, Wang T, et al. The gut microbiota as an environmental factor that regulates fat storage. Proc Natl Acad Sci U S A 2004;101:15718–23.
15. Guarner F, Malagelada JR. Gut flora in health and disease. Lancet 2003;361: 512–9.
16. Rakoff-Nahoum S, Paglino J, Eslami-Varzaneh F, et al. Recognition of commensal microflora by toll-like receptors is required for intestinal homeostasis. Cell 2004; 118:229–41.
17. Round JL, Mazmanian SK. The gut microbiota shapes intestinal immune responses during health and disease. Nat Rev Immunol 2009;9:313–23.
18. Abreu MT. Toll-like receptor signalling in the intestinal epithelium: how bacterial recognition shapes intestinal function. Nat Rev Immunol 2010;10:131–44.
19. Kosloske AM. Epidemiology of necrotizing enterocolitis. Acta Paediatr Suppl 1994;396:2–7.
20. Gewolb IH, Schwalbe RS, Taciak VL, et al. Stool microflora in extremely low birth-weight infants. Arch Dis Child Fetal Neonatal Ed 1999;80:F167–73.
21. Cotten CM, Taylor S, Stoll B, et al. Prolonged duration of initial empirical antibiotic treatment is associated with increased rates of necrotizing enterocolitis and death for extremely low birth weight infants. Pediatrics 2009;123:58–66.
22. Kenyon S, Boulvain M, Neilson J. Antibiotics for preterm premature rupture of membranes. Cochrane Database Syst Rev 2001;(8):CD001058.
23. Kuppala VS, Meinzen-Derr J, Morrow AL, et al. Prolonged initial empirical antibiotic treatment is associated with adverse outcomes in premature infants. J Pediatr 2011;159:720–5.
24. Alexander VN, Northrup V, Bizzarro MJ. Antibiotic exposure in the newborn intensive care unit and the risk of necrotizing enterocolitis. J Pediatr 2011;159:392–7.
25. Penders J, Thijs C, Vink C, et al. Factors influencing the composition of the intestinal microbiota in early infancy. Pediatrics 2006;118:511–21.
26. Westerbeek EA, van den Berg A, Lafeber HN, et al. The intestinal bacterial colonisation in preterm infants: a review of the literature. Clin Nutr 2006;25:361–8.
27. Goldmann DA, Leclair J, Macone A. Bacterial colonization of neonates admitted to an intensive care environment. J Pediatr 1978;93:288–93.
28. Mshvildadze M, Neu J. The infant intestinal microbiome: friend or foe? Early Hum Dev 2010;86(Suppl 1):67–71.
29. Mshvildadze M, Neu J, Shuster J, et al. Intestinal microbial ecology in premature infants assessed with non-culture-based techniques. J Pediatr 2010;156: 20–5.
30. Morowitz MJ, Poroyko V, Caplan M, et al. Redefining the role of intestinal microbes in the pathogenesis of necrotizing enterocolitis. Pediatrics 2010; 125(4):777–85.
31. Teitelbaum JE, Walker WA. Nutritional impact of pre- and probiotics as protective gastrointestinal organisms. Annu Rev Nutr 2002;22:107–38.
32. Mack DR, Lebel S. Role of probiotics in the modulation of intestinal infections and inflammation. Curr Opin Gastroenterol 2004;20:22–6.
33. Sartor RB. Therapeutic manipulation of the enteric microflora in inflammatory bowel diseases: antibiotics, probiotics, and prebiotics. Gastroenterology 2004; 126:1620–33.
34. Neish AS, Gewirtz AT, Zeng H, et al. Prokaryotic regulation of epithelial responses by inhibition of IkappaB-alpha ubiquitination. Science 2000;289:1560–3.
35. Lin PW, Nasr TR, Berardinelli AJ, et al. The probiotic Lactobacillus GG may augment intestinal host defense by regulating apoptosis and promoting cytoprotective responses in the developing murine gut. Pediatr Res 2008;64:511–6.

36. Khailova L, Mount Patrick SK, Arganbright KM, et al. *Bifidobacterium bifidum* reduces apoptosis in the intestinal epithelium in necrotizing enterocolitis. Am J Physiol Gastrointest Liver Physiol 2010;299:G1118–27.
37. Lin PW, Myers LE, Ray L, et al. *Lactobacillus rhamnosus* blocks inflammatory signaling in vivo via reactive oxygen species generation. Free Radic Biol Med 2009;47:1205–11.
38. Kumar A, Wu H, Collier-Hyams LS, et al. Commensal bacteria modulate cullin-dependent signaling via generation of reactive oxygen species. EMBO J 2007; 26:4457–66.
39. Patel RM, Myers LS, Kurundkar AR, et al. Probiotic bacteria induce maturation of intestinal claudin 3 expression and barrier function. Am J Pathol 2012;180: 626–35.
40. Khailova L, Dvorak K, Arganbright KM, et al. *Bifidobacterium bifidum* improves intestinal integrity in a rat model of necrotizing enterocolitis. Am J Physiol Gastrointest Liver Physiol 2009;297:G940–9.
41. Li N, Russell WM, Douglas-escobar M, et al. Live and heat-killed *Lactobacillus rhamnosus* GG: effects on proinflammatory and anti-inflammatory cytokines/chemokines in gastrostomy-fed infant rats. Pediatr Res 2009;66:203–7.
42. Ouwehand AC, Derrien M, de Vos W, et al. Prebiotics and other microbial substrates for gut functionality. Curr Opin Biotechnol 2005;16:212–7.
43. Ghisolfi J. Dietary fibre and prebiotics in infant formulas. Proc Nutr Soc 2003;62: 183–5.
44. Braegger C, Chmielewska A, Decsi T, et al. Supplementation of infant formula with probiotics and/or prebiotics: a systematic review and comment by the ESPGHAN committee on nutrition. J Pediatr Gastroenterol Nutr 2011;52:238–50.
45. Knol J, Boehm G, Lidestri M, et al. Increase of faecal bifidobacteria due to dietary oligosaccharides induces a reduction of clinically relevant pathogen germs in the faeces of formula-fed preterm infants. Acta Paediatr Suppl 2005;94:31–3.
46. Boehm G, Lidestri M, Casetta P, et al. Supplementation of a bovine milk formula with an oligosaccharide mixture increases counts of faecal bifidobacteria in preterm infants. Arch Dis Child Fetal Neonatal Ed 2002;86:F178–81.
47. Kapiki A, Costalos C, Oikonomidou C, et al. The effect of a fructo-oligosaccharide supplemented formula on gut flora of preterm infants. Early Hum Dev 2007;83: 335–9.
48. Underwood MA, Salzman NH, Bennett SH, et al. A randomized placebo-controlled comparison of 2 prebiotic/probiotic combinations in preterm infants: impact on weight gain, intestinal microbiota, and fecal short-chain fatty acids. J Pediatr Gastroenterol Nutr 2009;48:216–25.
49. Indrio F, Riezzo G, Raimondi F, et al. Effects of probiotic and prebiotic on gastrointestinal motility in newborns. J Physiol Pharmacol 2009;60(Suppl 6):27–31.
50. Indrio F, Riezzo G, Raimondi F, et al. Prebiotics improve gastric motility and gastric electrical activity in preterm newborns. J Pediatr Gastroenterol Nutr 2009;49:258–61.
51. Labayen I, Forga L, Gonzalez A, et al. Relationship between lactose digestion, gastrointestinal transit time and symptoms in lactose malabsorbers after dairy consumption. Aliment Pharmacol Ther 2001;15:543–9.
52. Boehm G, Stahl B, Jelinek J, et al. Prebiotic carbohydrates in human milk and formulas. Acta Paediatr Suppl 2005;94:18–21.
53. Fanaro S, Boehm G, Garssen J, et al. Galacto-oligosaccharides and long-chain fructo-oligosaccharides as prebiotics in infant formulas: a review. Acta Paediatr Suppl 2005;94:22–6.

54. Tsukahara T, Iwasaki Y, Nakayama K, et al. Stimulation of butyrate production in the large intestine of weaning piglets by dietary fructooligosaccharides and its influence on the histological variables of the large intestinal mucosa. J Nutr Sci Vitaminol (Tokyo) 2003;49:414–21.
55. Bartholome AL, Albin DM, Baker DH, et al. Supplementation of total parenteral nutrition with butyrate acutely increases structural aspects of intestinal adaptation after an 80% jejunoileal resection in neonatal piglets. JPEN J Parenter Enteral Nutr 2004;28:210–22 [discussion: 22–3].
56. Kanauchi O, Andoh A, Iwanaga T, et al. Germinated barley foodstuffs attenuate colonic mucosal damage and mucosal nuclear factor kappa B activity in a spontaneous colitis model. J Gastroenterol Hepatol 1999;14:1173–9.
57. Yin L, Laevsky G, Giardina C. Butyrate suppression of colonocyte NF-kappa B activation and cellular proteasome activity. J Biol Chem 2001;276:44641–6.
58. Venkatraman A, Ramakrishna BS, Shaji RV, et al. Amelioration of dextran sulfate colitis by butyrate: role of heat shock protein 70 and NF-kappaB. Am J Physiol Gastrointest Liver Physiol 2003;285:G177–84.
59. Kumar A, Wu H, Collier-Hyams LS, et al. The bacterial fermentation product butyrate influences epithelial signaling via reactive oxygen species-mediated changes in cullin-1 neddylation. J Immunol 2009;182:538–46.
60. Avivi-Green C, Polak-Charcon S, Madar Z, et al. Apoptosis cascade proteins are regulated in vivo by high intracolonic butyrate concentration: correlation with colon cancer inhibition. Oncol Res 2000;12:83–95.
61. Mentschel J, Claus R. Increased butyrate formation in the pig colon by feeding raw potato starch leads to a reduction of colonocyte apoptosis and a shift to the stem cell compartment. Metabolism 2003;52:1400–5.
62. Scheppach W, Weiler F. The butyrate story: old wine in new bottles? Curr Opin Clin Nutr Metab Care 2004;7:563–7.
63. Wang Q, Dong J, Zhu Y. Probiotic supplement reduces risk of necrotizing enterocolitis and mortality in preterm very low-birth-weight infants: an updated meta-analysis of 20 randomized, controlled trials. J Pediatr Surg 2012;47:241–8.
64. Sherman PM, Cabana M, Gibson GR, et al. Potential roles and clinical utility of prebiotics in newborns, infants, and children: proceedings from a global prebiotic summit meeting, New York City, June 27-28, 2008. J Pediatr 2009;155:S61–70.
65. Srinivasjois R, Rao S, Patole S. Prebiotic supplementation of formula in preterm neonates: a systematic review and meta-analysis of randomised controlled trials. Clin Nutr 2009;28:237–42.
66. Deshpande G, Rao S, Patole S, et al. Updated meta-analysis of probiotics for preventing necrotizing enterocolitis in preterm neonates. Pediatrics 2010;125:921–30.
67. Manzoni P, Rinaldi M, Cattani S, et al. Bovine lactoferrin supplementation for prevention of late-onset sepsis in very low-birth-weight neonates: a randomized trial. JAMA 2009;302:1421–8.
68. Samanta M, Sarkar M, Ghosh P, et al. Prophylactic probiotics for prevention of necrotizing enterocolitis in very low birth weight newborns. J Trop Pediatr 2009;55:128–31.
69. Lin HC, Hsu CH, Chen HL, et al. Oral probiotics prevent necrotizing enterocolitis in very low birth weight preterm infants: a multicenter, randomized, controlled trial. Pediatrics 2008;122:693–700.
70. Ohishi A, Takahashi S, Ito Y, et al. Bifidobacterium septicemia associated with postoperative probiotic therapy in a neonate with omphalocele. J Pediatr 2010;156:679–81.

71. Guenther K, Straube E, Pfister W, et al. Severe sepsis after probiotic treatment with *Escherichia coli* NISSLE 1917. Pediatr Infect Dis J 2010;29:188–9.
72. Land MH, Rouster-Stevens K, Woods CR, et al. Lactobacillus sepsis associated with probiotic therapy. Pediatrics 2005;115:178–81.
73. Thomas DW, Greer FR. Probiotics and prebiotics in pediatrics. Pediatrics 2010; 126:1217–31.
74. Claud EC, Lu L, Anton PM, et al. Developmentally regulated IkappaB expression in intestinal epithelium and susceptibility to flagellin-induced inflammation. Proc Natl Acad Sci U S A 2004;101:7404–8.
75. Nanthakumar NN, Fusunyan RD, Sanderson I, et al. Inflammation in the developing human intestine: a possible pathophysiologic contribution to necrotizing enterocolitis. Proc Natl Acad Sci U S A 2000;97:6043–8.
76. Sharma R, Tepas JJ 3rd, Hudak ML, et al. Neonatal gut barrier and multiple organ failure: role of endotoxin and proinflammatory cytokines in sepsis and necrotizing enterocolitis. J Pediatr Surg 2007;42:454–61.
77. van Elburg RM, Fetter WP, Bunkers CM, et al. Intestinal permeability in relation to birth weight and gestational and postnatal age. Arch Dis Child Fetal Neonatal Ed 2003;88:F52–5.
78. Thuijls G, Derikx JP, van Wijck K, et al. Non-invasive markers for early diagnosis and determination of the severity of necrotizing enterocolitis. Ann Surg 2010;251: 1174–80.
79. Nowicki PT, Nankervis CA. The role of the circulation in the pathogenesis of necrotizing enterocolitis. Clin Perinatol 1994;21:219–34.
80. Berseth CL. Gestational evolution of small intestine motility in preterm and term infants. J Pediatr 1989;115:646–51.
81. Anderson DM, Kliegman RM. The relationship of neonatal alimentation practices to the occurrence of endemic necrotizing enterocolitis. Am J Perinatol 1991;8: 62–7.
82. Berseth CL, Bisquera JA, Paje VU. Prolonging small feeding volumes early in life decreases the incidence of necrotizing enterocolitis in very low birth weight infants. Pediatrics 2003;111:529–34.
83. Lucas A, Cole TJ. Breast milk and neonatal necrotising enterocolitis. Lancet 1990; 336:1519–23.
84. Ip S, Chung M, Raman G, et al. Breastfeeding and maternal and infant health outcomes in developed countries. Evid Rep Technol Assess (Full Rep) 2007;(153): 1–186.
85. Claud EC, Walker WA. Hypothesis: inappropriate colonization of the premature intestine can cause neonatal necrotizing enterocolitis. FASEB J 2001;15:1398–403.
86. Kitajima H, Sumida Y, Tanaka R, et al. Early administration of *Bifidobacterium breve* to preterm infants: randomised controlled trial. Arch Dis Child Fetal Neonatal Ed 1997;76:F101–7.
87. Dani C, Biadaioli R, Bertini G, et al. Probiotics feeding in prevention of urinary tract infection, bacterial sepsis and necrotizing enterocolitis in preterm infants. A prospective double-blind study. Biol Neonate 2002;82:103–8.
88. Costalos C, Skouteri V, Gounaris A, et al. Enteral feeding of premature infants with *Saccharomyces boulardii*. Early Hum Dev 2003;74:89–96.
89. Bin-Nun A, Bromiker R, Wilschanski M, et al. Oral probiotics prevent necrotizing enterocolitis in very low birth weight neonates. J Pediatr 2005;147:192–6.
90. Lin HC, Su BH, Chen AC, et al. Oral probiotics reduce the incidence and severity of necrotizing enterocolitis in very low birth weight infants. Pediatrics 2005;115:1–4.

91. Manzoni P, Mostert M, Leonessa ML, et al. Oral supplementation with *Lactobacillus casei* subspecies *rhamnosus* prevents enteric colonization by Candida species in preterm neonates: a randomized study. Clin Infect Dis 2006;42: 1735–42.

92. Mohan R, Koebnick C, Schildt J, et al. Effects of *Bifidobacterium lactis* Bb12 supplementation on intestinal microbiota of preterm infants: a double-blind, placebo-controlled, randomized study. J Clin Microbiol 2006;44:4025–31.

93. Stratiki Z, Costalos C, Sevastiadou S, et al. The effect of a bifidobacter supplemented bovine milk on intestinal permeability of preterm infants. Early Hum Dev 2007;83:575–9.

94. Rouge C, Piloquet H, Butel MJ, et al. Oral supplementation with probiotics in very-low-birth-weight preterm infants: a randomized, double-blind, placebo-controlled trial. Am J Clin Nutr 2009;89:1828–35.

95. Mihatsch WA, Vossbeck S, Eikmanns B, et al. Effect of *Bifidobacterium lactis* on the incidence of nosocomial infections in very-low-birth-weight infants: a randomized controlled trial. Neonatology 2010;98:156–63.

96. Braga TD, da Silva GA, de Lira PI, et al. Efficacy of *Bifidobacterium breve* and *Lactobacillus casei* oral supplementation on necrotizing enterocolitis in very-low-birth-weight preterm infants: a double-blind, randomized, controlled trial. Am J Clin Nutr 2011;93:81–6.

97. Sari FN, Dizdar EA, Oguz S, et al. Oral probiotics: lactobacillus sporogenes for prevention of necrotizing enterocolitis in very low-birth weight infants: a randomized, controlled trial. Eur J Clin Nutr 2011;65:434–9.

98. Fernandez-Carrocera LA, Solis-Herrera A, Cabanillas-Ayon M, et al. Double-blind, randomised clinical assay to evaluate the efficacy of probiotics in preterm newborns weighing less than 1500 g in the prevention of necrotising enterocolitis. Arch Dis Child Fetal Neonatal Ed 2013;98(1):F5–9.

A Clinical Perspective of Necrotizing Enterocolitis
Past, Present, and Future

Renu Sharma, MD[a],*, Mark Lawrence Hudak, MD[b]

KEYWORDS

- Necrotizing enterocolitis • Isolated intestinal perforation • Peritoneal drainage
- Microecology • Inflammation

KEY POINTS

- There is an inverse relationship between postmenstrual age (PMA) at birth and risk of NEC. It is less common in term or late preterm infants.
- Intestinal immaturity, aggressive feedings, and inflammatory response to interactions between intestinal epithelial barrier and luminal microbes are key contributors to NEC.
- At an early stage, NEC is difficult to differentiate from sepsis. Intramural gas or pneumatosis and portal venous gas are pathognomonic signs of NEC.
- Pneumoperitoneum, a sign of intestinal perforation and signs of intestinal gangrene including severe metabolic acidosis, persistent and severe thrombocytopenia, adynamic dilated intestinal loops require surgical intervention.
- Research focused at identifying infants at increased risk of NEC combined with techniques aimed at early diagnosis, should decrease incidence and mortality of NEC.

FROM THE NINETEENTH TO THE TWENTY-FIRST CENTURY

In 1823, Charles Billard described what could be argued to be the first case report of necrotizing enterocolitis (NEC) as *gangrenous enterocolitis* in a small weak infant with infection, inflammation, and necrosis of the gastrointestinal tract (GIT).[1] This report was followed in 1850 by a publication of a series of 25 term and preterm

This work was supported by the National Institute of Child Health and Human Development grant number RO1 HD 059143.

The authors have no conflict of interest to declare.

[a] Division of Neonatology, Department of Pediatrics, University of Florida College of Medicine at Jacksonville, 655 West 8th Street, Jacksonville, FL 32209, USA; [b] Division of Neonatology, Department of Pediatrics, University of Florida College of Medicine at Jacksonville, 653-1 West 8th Street, LRC, 3rd Floor, Box L-16, Jacksonville, FL 32209, USA

* Corresponding author. Division of Neonatology, University of Florida at Jacksonville, 655 West 8th Street, Jacksonville, FL 32209.

E-mail address: renu.sharma@jax.ufl.edu

infants who presented with nonspecific clinical signs that rapidly progressed and resulted in death and who demonstrated similar pathologic findings on postmortem examinations.[1] With the advent of special care nurseries in Europe during the first part of the twentieth century, the clinical description of NEC began to emerge; by the latter half, this disease was widely recognized as the most serious gastrointestinal emergency in intensive care nurseries worldwide. In 1965, Mizrahi and colleagues[2] first used the term *necrotizing enterocolitis* to describe a clinical syndrome consisting of vomiting, abdominal distension, shock, and intestinal hemorrhage and perforation. The initial surgical approach to this disease was formulated by Touloukian[3] and Santulli and colleagues[4] in the 1970s. In 1978, Bell and colleagues[5] classified NEC into 3 stages based on the severity of the clinical presentation and recommended treatment strategies. Despite incremental advances in our understanding of the clinical presentation and pathophysiology of NEC, universal prevention of this serious and often fatal disease continues to elude us even in the twenty-first century.

WHO IS AT RISK? HOW PREVALENT IT IS?

NEC primarily affects premature infants. It is less common in term and late preterm infants.[6,7] Only 7% to 15% of all NEC cases occur in term or late preterm infants (**Fig. 1A**). The age of onset is inversely related to the postmenstrual age (PMA) at birth (see **Fig. 1B**).[7] In term infants, NEC is commonly associated with congenital heart diseases, such as hypoplastic left heart syndrome and coarctation of the aorta, which result in intestinal hypoxia and/or hypoperfusion.[8] NEC has also been associated with other anomalies, including aganglionosis[9] and gastroschisis.[10] More than 85% of all NEC cases occur in very low birth weight (VLBW) infants (<1500 g) or in very premature (VP) infants (<32 weeks of PMA).[11]

The prevalence of NEC varies among centers. Multicenter and large population-based studies demonstrate that it is prevalent in 7% to 11% of VLBW infants.[11–13] The National Institute of Child Health (NICHD) Neonatal Research Network (NRN) study reported a 7% prevalence rate of NEC in a population of 11,072 VLBW infants during 1999 to 2001.[14] The Vermont Oxford Network also reported a similar prevalence rate (7.4%) in 71,808 VLBW infants during a study period from 2005 to 2006.[15] A concurrent NICHD-NRN study from 2003 to 2007 found that the prevalence of NEC remained high (11%) among VP infants (born at 22–28 weeks of PMA, birth weight 401–1500 g).[13] The prevalence of NEC seems to be less in Europe and Canada. A recent Swedish study found that 5.8% of infants born before 27 weeks of PMA developed NEC among a cohort of 638 infants.[16] A Swiss neonatal network study reported that only 3% to 4% of infants born at less than 32 weeks of PMA during 2000 to 2004 developed NEC.[17] The Canadian Neonatal Network documented that 5.1% of infants born earlier than 33 weeks of PMA developed NEC during 2003 to 2008 in a population of 16,669 infants.[18] Despite the improvement in survival of VLBW infants, neonatal NEC remains quite prevalent in the United States (0.3–2.4 infants per 1000 live births).[19]

The overall mortality for NEC ranges from 20% to 40% but approaches 100% in infants with the most severe form of the disease.[12,15,20] Boys have a higher risk of death than girls.[12] Earlier studies have reported a slight increase in the prevalence of NEC among African American and male infants, but more recent studies have failed to verify these observations.[12] Because NEC affects 2% to 5% of all NICU admissions and causes serious morbidity, NEC continues to impose a heavy burden on the neonatal population.[19]

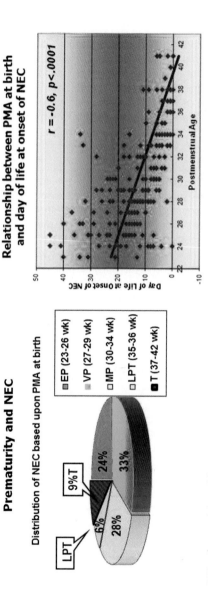

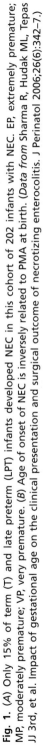

A

Prematurity and NEC

Distribution of NEC based upon PMA at birth

- ■ EP (23-26 wk)
- ▨ VP (27-29 wk)
- □ MP (30-34 wk)
- ▨ LPT (35-36 wk)
- ■ T (37-42 wk)

B

Relationship between PMA at birth and day of life at onset of NEC

$r = -0.6, p < .0001$

Postmenstrual Age

Day of Life at Onset of NEC

Fig. 1. (A) Only 15% of term (T) and late preterm (LPT) infants developed NEC in this cohort of 202 infants with NEC. EP, extremely premature; MP, moderately premature; VP, very premature. (B) Age of onset of NEC is inversely related to PMA at birth. (*Data from* Sharma R, Hudak ML, Tepas JJ 3rd, et al. Impact of gestational age on the clinical presentation and surgical outcome of necrotizing enterocolitis. J Perinatol 2006;26(6):342–7.)

WHAT CAUSES NEC? HOW DOES IT HAPPEN?

The pathophysiology of NEC in VP infants is not completely elucidated. Compared with NEC in term and late preterm infants in whom hypoxia-ischemia is a common precursor, recent advances in our understanding of NEC at the molecular level suggest that an inflammatory response in VP infants plays the inciting or dominant role in the pathogenesis of NEC.[21,22] Previously held beliefs that low Apgar scores,[23] umbilical catheterizations, episodes of apnea and bradycardia, respiratory distress syndrome, anemia, hypothermia, hypoxic-ischemic events,[24–27] hypotension, and the use of vasoactive agents such as Indocin[25] and pressors are important contributing causes of NEC in premature infants have not been supported by large epidemiologic and more recent clinical studies.[6] Although hemorrhagic-ischemic necrosis is the terminal manifestation of NEC in premature infants, the interaction among milk substrate, microbes, and the immature host immunologic system is now thought to be key in initiating the pathogenesis of NEC (**Fig. 2**).[22]

Aggressive Feeding

In premature infants, aggressive feeding may cause stasis of milk substrate in the lumen of the GIT because of dysmotility.[28] Stasis can lead to intestinal dilatation with fluid and gas and possibly to impairment of the intestinal epithelial barrier (IEB).[29–31] The development of endotoxemia in stable premature infants after feeding and evidence from other studies support that the IEB of premature infants is leakier compared with that of more mature infants.[31–34] Intestinal dilatation in the presence of abnormal microbial colonization (dysbiosis) can distort normal signal transduction (crosstalk) across the IEB and alter the normal message of growth and repair of enterocytes to one that instead produces excessive inflammation, apoptosis, and necrosis (**Fig. 3**).[32,34,35]

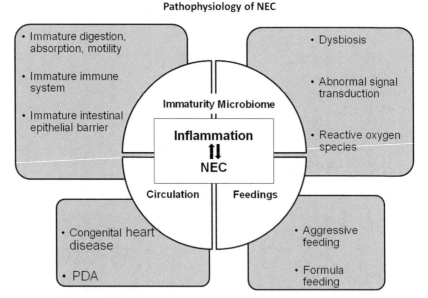

Fig. 2. Pathophysiology of NEC.

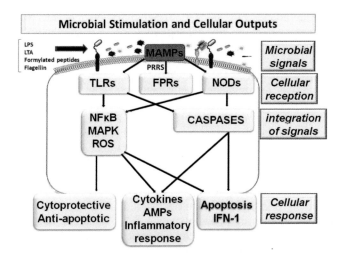

Fig. 3. Microbial components, such as lipopolysaccharides (LPS), lipoteichoic acid (LTA), formylated peptides, and flagellin, serve as microbial-associated molecular patterns (MAMPs) and signal pattern recognition receptors (PRRs), including toll-like receptors (TLRs), formylated peptide receptors (FPRs), or nucleotide-binding oligomerization domain-like receptors (NODs). Integration of these signals evokes cellular outputs based on the initial perception of the triggering organism. Output can be a protective response to commensal microbiota, an inflammatory response to pathogenic organisms, or it can trigger apoptosis. (*Adapted from* Sharma R, Young C, Neu J. Molecular modulation of intestinal epithelial barrier: contribution of microbiota. J Biomed Biotechnol 2010;2010:305879; with permission.)

Transfusion and NEC

In recent years, several reports have attempted to establish a causal relationship between blood transfusion (BT) and NEC.[36–42] These studies propose that BT for anemia of prematurity in relatively stable growing premature infants increases the risk of late-onset NEC. The authors think that additional prospective reports that use a more robust design and analysis are needed before a causative relationship can be accepted because of the weaknesses in study designs of these investigations (eg, failure to include all BT, retrospective nature of data collection, lack of appropriate case-control matching, and failure to control for confounding variables). A recently completed prospective, matched, case-control investigation that used robust methodology does not substantiate an association between BT and NEC.

Microbial Mucosal Interactions and NEC

At the mucosal surface, signals from microbial ligands like endotoxin (synonymous with lipopolysaccharide [LPS]), flagellin, lipoteichoic acid, peptidoglycans, and formylated peptides are communicated through a sophisticated process (crosstalk) to appropriate epithelial receptors specific for that ligand referred to as pattern recognition receptors (PRRs), including Toll-like receptors (TLRs), formylated peptide receptors, and nucleotide-binding oligomerization domains.[35] Activation of these PRRs initiates regulatory pathways, including mitogen-activated protein kinase, nuclear factor κB (NFκB), and caspase-dependent pathways (see **Fig. 3**).[22,29,35,43–45] These interrelated complex pathways determine mucosal and submucosal responses. Based on the perception of interrelated signals, the response can be cytoprotective (ie, promoting growth and repair) or it can be destructive if apoptosis or inflammatory responses is triggered (see **Fig. 3**).[22,35,44] The terminal event in NEC is hemorrhagic-ischemic necrosis, which is the consequence of a dysregulated inflammatory response mediated by endogenous factors that include platelet-activating factor (PAF), proinflammatory cytokines (such as tumor necrosis factor-α, interleukins 1 & 6 [IL-1, IL-6]), chemokines (MIP-2/CXCL2), NF-κB, and the complement system.[29]

Because of the relative immaturity of key gastrointestinal functions, such as digestion, absorption, motility, and abnormalities in immune responses, a premature newborn is exquisitely vulnerable to gastrointestinal injury.[46] The cellular response to signal transduction as described earlier is orchestrated by the innate immune system in mucosa and submucosa.[45,47] Microbial interaction with intestinal epithelium (PRRS) signals tissue-specific functions, such as T-cell expansion and elaboration of cytokines and chemokines. Normally after birth, exposure to LPS downregulates IL-1 receptor associated kinase 1 (IRAK), an intermediary for epithelial TLR4 signaling, and promotes tolerance to LPS.[19,22,43] This postnatal adaptation helps to achieve host-microbe homeostasis with microbial tolerance.[22,44] Premature infants are exposed shortly after birth to a massive microbial antigenic challenge that may be distorted by frequent and prolonged use of antibiotics. As a result, the GIT of premature infants gravitates toward mounting an inflammatory response rather than establishing tolerance (T-helper-1 response).[30,35,47] The premature infant seems to mimic a response that is similar to the immune-naïve response demonstrated by the fetus, which is characterized by hyper-responsiveness to LPS.[22,48]

Intestinal colonization with commensal *Bifidobacterium* and *Lactobacillus* species reduces the risk of NEC.[49,50] The frequent and prolonged use of antibiotics results in an overgrowth of potentially pathogenic species.[51] Distortion of intestinal microecology by exposure to broad-spectrum antibiotics may result in colonization with inflammogenic microbial consortia that are more likely to direct the immune repertoire in the direction of an inflammatory response, thereby increasing the risk for NEC.[51,52] Metagenomic studies indicate that intestinal microecology during the early postnatal period greatly influences the evolution of immune health.[53,54] Infants who later develop NEC show evidence for a dysbiotic microecology before the diagnosis of NEC.[55] A recent clinical study found that exposure to broad-spectrum antibiotics for more than 10 days increased the risk of NEC by nearly threefold.[51]

Recent advances in the proteomics and microecology pertinent to NEC strongly suggest that a distorted innate-immune response of premature infants increases the vulnerability to NEC.[22,55] Glucocorticoid-mediated maturation of the IEB has been shown to protect against NEC and to blunt the inflammatory response seen in NEC.[46,48,56,57] Furthermore, the vulnerability to NEC is not unique to premature neonates, it is also seen in the older immune-compromised population.[58–60] A NEC-like illness has been described in the geriatric population and in patients with human immunodeficiency virus.[56,58]

Hypoxic-Ischemic Mechanisms

Under normal conditions, a state of high intestinal blood flow and low resting vascular resistance is maintained by nitric oxide.[26] Impaired endothelial function or elaboration of proinflammatory mediators may alter the balance between vasoconstriction (as mediated by endothelin-1) and vasodilatation (as mediated by nitric oxide) and lead to a relatively ischemic state. In animal models of hypoxia-ischemia, derangements of intestinal microcirculation develop at the premucosal arteriolar inflow location with a distinct stop-and-go pattern consistent with severe vascular dysfunction.[61] Levels of inflammatory mediators increase markedly in real-time animal models of NEC.[61–63] The elaboration of inflammatory mediators (eg, PAF) early in the pathogenesis of NEC may have important secondary effects on local circulation that contribute to the development of the intestinal necrosis.[19,27,43,63–65]

Infectious Agents

Despite 4 decades of exhaustive search, no consistent single microbial species has been isolated from infants with NEC.[66] *Enterobacteriaceae* sp are the most common, followed by *Staphylococcus* sp and *Clostridium* sp.[19,67–70] Outbreaks of NEC linked to consumption of formula contaminated by *Enterobacter sakazakii* and breast milk contaminated by *Staphylococci* have occurred.[69–71] Although bacteria are most commonly associated with NEC, several enteric viruses (rotavirus, echovirus, coronavirus, torovirus, norovirus [NoV]) and *Candida* sp have also been described.[72–80]

Generally, NEC occurs sporadically but may also occur in clusters or outbreaks.[81] Temporal clustering of such outbreaks and their cessation with the implementation of infection control measures supports an association of these outbreaks with a single transmissible agent during a given outbreak.[82,83] As cited earlier, varieties of organisms, including bacteria and viruses, have been linked to outbreaks of NEC. Among viruses, NoV, astrovirus, torovirus, coronavirus, and rotavirus have been linked with outbreaks of hemorrhagic gastroenteritis and necrotizing enterocolitis.[75,79,84–86] In a recent study, compared with infants with rotavirus or norovirus enteritis, infants with astrovirus were more likely to develop NEC and the systemic inflammatory response syndrome.[87]

Viral enterotoxin, such as the nonstructural protein (NSP4) of rotavirus, stimulates a secretory response that is Ca^{++} dependent that results in watery diarrhea in mature infants but hemorrhagic enteritis or NEC in premature infants.[75,88] This viral enterotoxin induces an age- and dose-dependent response.[88] NSP4 increases paracellular permeability and alters the integrity of the IEB. It binds with caveolin-1 (scaffolding protein) and alters tight junction assembly.[89–91] Consequently, a weakened IEB permits the translocation of microbes and the initiation of endotoxemia and the inflammatory response characteristic of NEC.[90]

Regardless of whether a pathogen can be identified during a local epidemic of NEC, implementation of infection control measures are effective in stopping the outbreak.[81,83,92,93]

HOW DOES IT PRESENT? HOW DO WE DIAGNOSE?
Clinical Signs

During the 1980s, investigators found that NEC occurred more commonly in preterm infants between 33 to 35 weeks of PMA.[94,95] More recent studies have found that a peak distribution of NEC occurs at 29 to 31 weeks of PMA (**Fig. 4**).[7] This shift to an earlier PMA may be a reflection of the current practice to introduce enteral feedings earlier compared with the delayed feeding practices of the 1980s.[94,95]

The clinical presentation of NEC can range from nonspecific signs that progress insidiously over several days to a fulminant onset of gastrointestinal signs, multiorgan system dysfunction, and shock over a few hours.[6] Early signs of NEC are nonspecific and may be indistinguishable from those of sepsis.[5,6,11,29,94,95] Clinical signs include both intestinal and systemic perturbations. Intestinal signs in early NEC can present as feeding intolerance that may manifest as increased prefeeding gastric residuals, emesis, abdominal distension, and bloody stools (hematochezia). Less commonly, when the stomach is involved, NEC can present as bloody emesis or a bloody gastric residual.[95,96] During the advanced stage of NEC, the abdomen may appear shiny, distended, and erythematous. Infants generally prefer to assume a frog-leg position (position of comfort, **Fig. 5**A) and are hyporesponsive.[6,94–96] On gentle palpation,

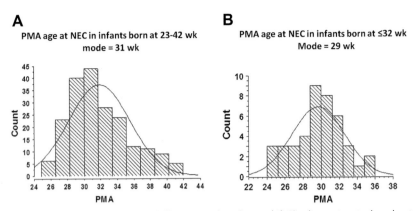

A

PMA age at NEC in infants born at 23-42 wk
mode = 31 wk

B

PMA age at NEC in infants born at ≤32 wk
Mode = 29 wk

Fig. 4. PMA at onset of NEC in 2 different study cohorts. (*A*) Single-center study cohort of 202 infants with NEC during 1991 to 2003 born at 23 to 42 weeks; NEC was most common at 31 weeks of PMA. (*B*) Multicenter study cohort of 42 infants with NEC during 2008 to 2012 born at 23 to 32 weeks; NEC occurred most commonly at 29 weeks of PMA.

the abdomen may feel firm, tense, and tender, and a tender mass may be palpable. Bowel perforation may cause the abdomen to appear blue or discolored.[6,94–96] An infant with a blue discolored abdomen secondary to isolated intestinal perforation may be indistinguishable from an infant with NEC. In a male infant, erythema or bluish discoloration of the scrotum may appear if peritoneal fluid from perforated bowel herniates into the scrotum (see **Fig. 5**B).

VP infants do not manifest tenderness and guarding unless NEC is advanced. Therefore, a high index of suspicion is required to establish a diagnosis of NEC if multiple subtle signs appear that produce a deviation from baseline clinical status.[6,7] NEC can also present with bloody stools (hematochezia) without any other initial signs, especially when NEC involves the distal colon. If the jejunum and terminal ileum are the predominant sites of NEC, then emesis, increased gastric residuals, and/or abdominal

Clinical findings

Shiny, distended, erythematous abdomen

Blue scrotum in infant with perforated NEC

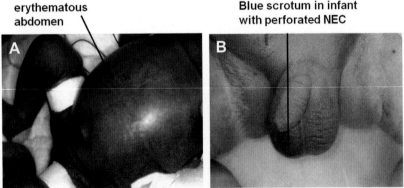

Fig. 5. (*A*) Shiny, distended, erythematous abdomen (*arrow*) of an infant with advanced NEC in frog-leg position. (*B*) Discolored scrotum (*arrow*) in an infant with perforated advanced NEC; no pneumoperitoneum was seen in abdominal radiographs.

distension are the more likely initial clinical signs.[97,98] Occult hematochezia diagnosed by a hemoccult test correlates poorly with NEC.[99]

Extremely premature infants with NEC are more likely to present with abdominal distension, ileus, and emesis. They are less likely to present with pneumatosis but are more likely to develop pneumoperitoneum compared with late-term or term infants (**Fig. 6**A, B). Observation of a lightly bile-stained gastric residual in VP infants, especially before any feeding, is common and normally resolves as gradual advancement of feeding volumes elicits improvement in intestinal motility. Consistent dark-green bilious gastric residual may indicate gastrointestinal obstruction and requires further investigation.[98]

Systemic signs include lethargy, hypotension, poor perfusion and pallor, increased episodes of apnea and bradycardia, worsening of respiratory function, temperature instability, tachycardia, hyperglycemia, or hypoglycemia.[95–98]

Abnormal laboratory tests include anemia, left shift of neutrophils, neutropenia, thrombocytopenia, metabolic acidosis, and hyponatremia.[98,100] In some instances, NEC may present as unexplained hyponatremia. Concurrent bacteremia and sepsis occurs in 40% to 60% of NEC cases.[97,98,100–102] Sepsis caused by gram-negative bacteria is more common.[97,102] Conversely, if an infant presents with sepsis caused by gram-negative bacteria and nonspecific intestinal and radiographic signs, there is a greater likelihood that NEC is the underlying cause of this illness.[102]

In 5% to 6% of cases, NEC may recur.[97,103] Recurrence is more likely if the initial episode of NEC was associated with congenital heart disease or with rotavirus. Recurrence can also occur with cow milk protein allergy.[104,105] However, NEC can recur after either medical or surgical NEC without specific risk factors.[97,103]

Radiographic Signs

Intramural gas or pneumatosis and portal venous gas are pathognomonic signs of NEC. They may appear even before clinical signs. The absence of these radiographic signs by no means confirms the absence of NEC. Pneumatosis is caused by gas within the

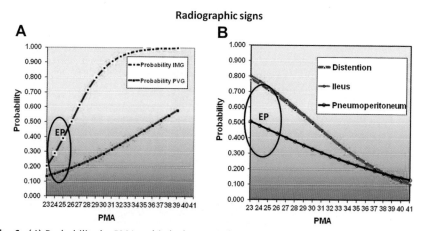

Fig. 6. (*A*) Probability by PMA at birth that an infant with NEC will present with intramural gas (IMG) or portal venous gas (PVG). There is less than 50% probability for an extremely premature (EP) infant to manifest IMG. (*B*) Radiographic signs that are more probable in infants with decreasing PMA. There is more than 50% probability that an EP infant will present with these signs. (*Adapted* and *Modified from* Sharma R, Hudak ML, Tepas JJ 3rd, et al. Impact of gestational age on the clinical presentation and surgical outcome of necrotizing enterocolitis. J Perinatol 2006;26(6):342–7; with permission.)

bowel wall and may appear linear (like railroad tracks) or circular if gas is subserosal or bubbly if gas is submucosal (**Fig. 7**).[106,107] Bubbly gas lucencies could also indicate air within intraluminal fecal material. Pneumatosis is more commonly seen in the right lower quadrant but it can be seen anywhere because necrosis may involve any section of bowel extending from the stomach to the rectum.[97,106,107] The amount of pneumatosis does not always relate to the severity of disease, and its disappearance does not necessarily imply pathologic or clinical improvement.[7,97,106,107] Other nonspecific but common abdominal radiographic findings include thickened bowel walls, dilated bowel loops, a paucity of bowel gas, and a fixed dilated loop (**Fig. 8**).[106,107] Inflamed, edematous, and hemorrhagic bowel wall may be separated from each other because of thickening of bowel wall and the normal sausage-like mosaic configuration may be lost. A persistent, fixed, dilated loop may indicate a necrotic bowel loop. Dilated, gas-filled loops in the central abdomen may indicate the presence of ascites or free peritoneal fluid because dilated bowel loops float (and migrate to the least dependent region of the abdomen) when peritoneal fluid is present.[106,107] A paucity of bowel gas may be associated with ileus and abdominal decompression. These nonspecific signs may not be diagnostic of NEC but nonetheless are non-reassuring and suspicious for NEC, thereby warranting immediate intervention and treatment implementation.[106,107]

Pneumatosis intestinalis can extend to the portal venous circulation and typically appear as curvilinear lucencies over the hepatic silhouette in a plain radiograph (see **Fig. 7**).[97] A pneumoperitoneum is diagnostic of a perforated viscus. In a supine position, it may appear as a rounded or oval extraluminal lucency beneath the upper anterior abdominal wall (**Fig. 9**). When there is a large pneumoperitoneum, it may outline

Pneumatosis and portal venous gas seen in plain radiographs and in abdominal CT

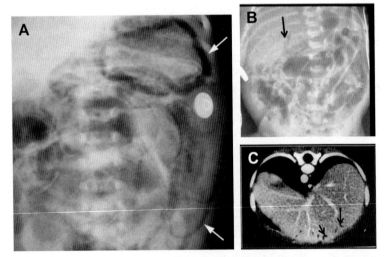

Fig. 7. (A) There is extensive pneumatosis (*arrows*); left upper arrow pointing at gastric pneumatosis. Pneumatosis is seen as multiple curvilinear radiolucencies in this plain radiograph. (B) Arrow pointing toward portal venous gas seen as curvilinear radiolucency over liver; distended bowel loops and diffuse pneumatosis is seen throughout. (C) Portal venous gas (*arrows*) is seen as lucencies in on computed tomography (CT) scan. ([A] *Adapted from* Epelman M, Daneman A, Navarro OM, et al. Necrotizing enterocolitis: review of state-of-the-art imaging findings with pathologic correlation. Radiographics 2007;27:285–305; with permission.)

Fixed dilated sausage
loops in NEC

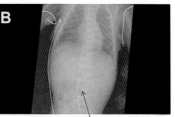

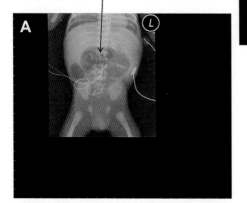

Fixed dilated
intestinal loops in
midline, remainder
gasless abdomen
indicating ascites

Fig. 8. (*A*) A dynamic loop in serial radiographs indicates intestinal necrosis. (*B*) Gasless abdomen with a few loops in midline indicates ascites (peritonitis) and intestinal necrosis.

Cross table lateral view of
pneumoperitoneum in NEC

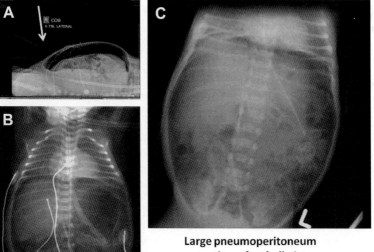

Large pneumoperitoneum
creating a football-sign

Large pneumoperitoneum creating
abdominal compartment syndrome

Fig. 9. (*A*) Cross-table lateral and (*B*) plain abdominal radiographs illustrating radiolucent pneumoperitoneum (*indicated by arrows*). (*C*) Another large pneumoperitoneum creating a football sign.

the falciform ligament giving it the appearance of a longitudinal strip of sutures in a football (American football and rugby but not soccer ball), leading to its designation as the football sign (see **Fig. 9**).[106,107] A cross-table lateral film may demonstrate small air collection just beneath the abdomen (see **Fig. 9**). A small pneumoperitoneum may be difficult to visualize on a single plain film. A left lateral decubitus film will allow free air to rise to the top over a nondependent surface, facilitating visualization of an abnormal lucency. A small amount of free air may present as a small triangular or a rectangular lucency and make a definitive diagnosis of free air difficult. Sometimes free air may present as a double-wall sign when the bowel loop is outlined and gas is present along serosal and mucosal surfaces.[106,107]

A nonionic water-soluble contrast study (typically, an upper gastrointestinal series followed by an enema) can be obtained in circumstances when anatomic gastrointestinal obstruction is suspected.[107] Hypertonic water-soluble agents are not routinely recommended because hypovolemia can result from a shift of fluid from the intravascular space to the intestinal lumen.[107]

Ultrasound

In situations when radiographic signs are nonspecific, the abdominal ultrasound (US) is another modality that can identify even small volumes of free gas. US is also the preferred modality for visualization of abdominal fluid and ascites. Thickness and echogenicity of the bowel wall and qualitative assessment of peristalsis can be visualized best by US color Doppler. It can also be used to assess arterial perfusion of the bowel wall (**Fig. 10**). Portal venous gas can be more readily seen using abdominal sonography than plain film.[107] Faingold and colleagues[108] used color Doppler sonography and demonstrated 100% sensitivity for free air and absent blood flow (necrotic gut) compared with 40% sensitivity by radiography. The use of computed tomography is not advocated for the diagnosis of NEC.[107]

MANAGEMENT
Medical

When an infant is suspected to have NEC, all enteral feedings and medications should be discontinued (**Fig. 11**). Prompt decompression of the GIT should be accomplished by the placement of a double-lumen gastric tube (large lumen for aspiration and small lumen for irrigation and venting) with the institution of low, constant suction. Aspirated volume should be replaced with intravenous Ringer lactate solution with extra potassium chloride that is lost in gastric output. It is crucial to ensure the patency of the tube. If the abdomen continues to distend despite ongoing continuous suction, the tube should be checked for proper placement and for blockage and nasal continuous positive airway pressure should be discontinued. Endotracheal intubation is preferred in infants who are deteriorating and have frequent episodes of apnea. Intravascular volume must be monitored rigorously to ensure adequate tissue perfusion and may be gauged by frequent assessment of serum electrolytes, hematocrit, and urinary output. As a rule of thumb, anticipation of third spacing in infants with NEC will require 1.5-fold maintenance fluid plus replacement of gastric output. Failure to maintain euvolemia and proper electrolyte repletion can result in shock with hypochloremia, hyponatremia, and hypokalemia. Parenteral nutrition should be started early with adequate protein (3.5–4.0 g/kg/d) to maintain positive nitrogen balance and to allow the repair of injured tissue.[6,46,109–111]

Strict implementation of infection control measures is critical. Following the culture of blood and urine, prompt initiation of treatment with appropriate broad-spectrum

Abdominal ultrasound in normal infant
and in infant with NEC

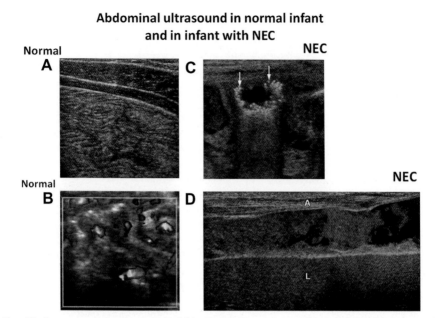

Fig. 10. Sonogram of normal bowel (*A, B*). (*A*) Normal non-distended bowel; echogenic markings represent mucosal interface with lumen, and hypoechoic linear bands represent the muscularis of the bowel wall. (*B*) Color Doppler image of non-distended normal bowel with color dots of blood flow in normal bowel. (*C*) Sonogram shows a distended loop with many pneumatoses seen as hyper-echoic bubbles (*arrows*). (*D*) Free intraperitoneal fluid in perforated NEC. Echogenic fluid between abdominal wall (A) and liver (L) is seen containing much debris, which is more indicative of bowel perforation than free fluid. (*Adapted from* Epelman M, Daneman A, Navarro OM, et al. Necrotizing enterocolitis: review of state-of-the-art imaging findings with pathologic correlation. Radiographics 2007;27:285–305; with permission.)

antibiotics based on known sensitivities of prevalent pathogens in the individual neonatal intensive care unit is vital. If surgical intervention is performed, peritoneal fluid and intestinal tissue should be sent for gram stain, culture, and sensitivity. The utility of a stool culture for bacteria in neonates has been questioned because fecal matter has many bacterial species. However, during outbreaks of NEC, attempts should be made to identify the infectious agent whenever possible. Usual regimens include ampicillin (or a cephalosporin) and gentamicin (or other aminoglycoside). The addition of a third antibiotic that provides anaerobic coverage (eg, clindamycin or metronidazole) is indicated when there is evidence of peritonitis or bowel perforation (see **Fig. 11**). Inflammation of the intestine and peritoneum is excruciatingly painful; therefore, attention to pain control and minimal handling during cares are integral parts of management.[6,46,109–111]

Hematocrit should be monitored and packed red cells should be provided to replace occult intestinal hemorrhage. Adjunctive treatment includes judicious correction of significant thrombocytopenia, coagulopathy, and metabolic acidosis. Abdominal girth should be measured frequently. A sudden increase in abdominal girth warrants an immediate abdominal radiograph to assess for a pneumoperitoneum. Co-management with pediatric surgeons is recommended when a diagnosis of NEC is strongly suspected or confirmed. In sick infants who are not improving despite supportive

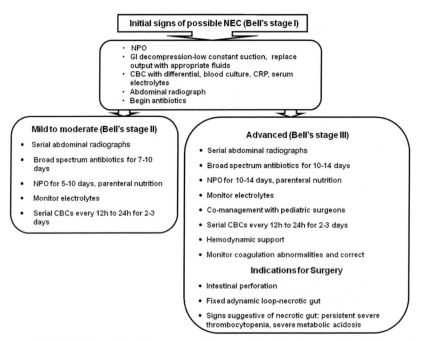

Fig. 11. Clinical decision algorithms. NPO, nil per os (nothing by mouth); CBC, complete blood cell count; CRP, C-reactive protein.

medical management and in whom NEC is suspected, consultation with a pediatric surgeon and radiologist may help to arrive at a specific diagnosis.[6,46,107,109–113]

In the most premature infants, a high index of suspicion is required to make a timely diagnosis of NEC because these infants are less likely to manifest tenderness and the pathognomonic radiographic findings of NEC.[7] By the time VP infants manifest tenderness or abdominal mass, NEC has usually progressed to an advanced stage.[7]

Surgical

Identification of a pneumoperitoneum caused by bowel perforation and the presence of necrotic bowel (either may be difficult to diagnose) are 2 absolute indications for surgical intervention. Severe and persistent metabolic acidosis and/or thrombocytopenia in conjunction with a lack of improvement with medical management strongly suggest the presence of necrotic bowel and warrants surgery (see **Fig. 11**).[7,97,100,102,110,112,113]

The timely diagnosis of bowel perforation or dead gut can be difficult in extremely premature infants with NEC.[7] A negative laparotomy is just as detrimental as failure to recognize perforation early in this group of patients.[107] Pneumoperitoneum can be missed in about 20% of cases of bowel perforation.[107] In such cases, the use of a 7-point scoring system using 7 components that quantitate the presence of metabolic derangement, in conjunction with an infant's ongoing evaluation by a pediatric surgeon, has been found to optimize the timing of the surgical intervention.[114] These metabolic derangements include severe metabolic acidosis, severe thrombocytopenia, hypotension, hyponatremia, neutropenia, left shift of neutrophils, and positive blood culture. It is recommended that this scoring system be used only as an adjunct to careful serial clinical and radiologic evaluation of infants.[108,110,114]

With respect to the type of surgery, primary peritoneal drainage (PPD) has emerged as an alternative to laparotomy in VP infants with bowel perforation.[100,115] Peritoneal drainage serves as a definitive treatment of some patients and as a temporizing measure for unstable sick infants until laparotomy can be performed after their stabilization.[115–119]

The choice of PPD or laparotomy as a primary surgical intervention has been argued for a decade.[116–118] In their review of only 2 randomized controlled trials, Rao and colleagues[116] report that there were no differences with respect to mortality and duration for total parenteral nutrition between the drainage and laparotomy. However, these studies did not distinguish between isolated perforation and NEC.[120] Neither of these two trials reached the recruitment target nor showed improved survival from PPD or laparotomy. One of these two trials [Necrotizing Enterocolitis Trial (NET) from the United Kingdom] found that 74% of infants initially treated with PPD required a rescue laparotomy. The second NICHD NRN trial did not encourage rescue laparotomy (which nonetheless was allowed) and did not distinguish NEC from isolated intestinal perforation (IIP).[117–119] This latter trial, conducted in extremely low birth weight infants (≤1000 g), found that laparotomy had an advantage over PPD with respect to the likelihood of survival and better neurodevelopmental outcome at 18 to 22 months of age.[120] Death or impairment occurred in 78% of the drainage group and in 66% of the laparotomy group.

The ability to accurately distinguish NEC from IIP is important when making a comparison between PPD and laparotomy because mortality associated with NEC is greater than with IIP.[120,121] A large, single-center, prospective study showed that bowel perforation in infants with severe NEC who were treated with primary laparotomy fared better than infants treated with a PPD.[100,121,122] Conversely, infants with IIP fared better with PPD. These investigators devised the 7-point metabolic derangement score and used it in conjunction with ultrasonography or contrast imaging to distinguish NEC from IIP.

Other traditional surgical procedures at laparotomy include debridement and the resection of clearly necrotic bowel and creation of an enterostomy.[113,120,121] Sometimes multiple excisions are needed to preserve bowel length. Viable ends of bowel are exteriorized as stomas with the distal end as a mucous fistula. Sometimes single stoma with a Hartmann pouch is created. In this procedure, a colostomy or ileostomy is created and the distal limb is closed by suturing it and placing it back in the peritoneal cavity as a temporary measure until the patient is ready for re-anastomosis.[110,113,123]

PATHOLOGY

Coagulation (hemorrhagic-ischemic) necrosis, inflammation, and bacterial overgrowth are salient features of the histopathology of NEC. Reparative tissue changes, such as epithelial regeneration, formation of granulation tissue, and fibrosis, are found in two-thirds of cases and provide evidence for a duration of tissue injury/reparation processes of at least several days.[124,125] Damage to the intestinal tract may range from mucosal injury to full-thickness necrosis with focal perforation. Gas bubbles (pneumatosis intestinalis) can be seen in mucosa, submucosa, and serosal surfaces (**Fig. 12**).[125] Although NEC can involve the gut from the stomach to the distal colon (NEC totalis), disease is most commonly found in the terminal ileum and ascending colon. Rotavirus-associated NEC most often involves the distal colon.[75] NEC can cause focal disease or manifest as multiple large diffuse necrotic areas alternating with patches of unaffected bowel. Serosal exudation without obvious perforation can also occur. In mild stages of NEC, intense congestion of superficial mucosa can result in focal necrosis of villous tips and epithelial sloughing into bowel lumen.[124,125]

Pathology of NEC

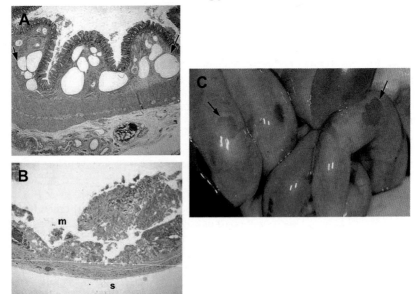

Fig. 12. (*A*) Histology of small bowel (original magnification × 100; hematoxylin-eosin stain) illustrating rounded large bubbles (*arrows*) of pneumatosis (intramural gas) in the submucosa. (*B*) At a more advanced stage, there is necrosis of mucosa, submucosa, and muscularis with intraluminal necrotic debris on the mucosal side (m), (original magnification × 100; hematoxylin-eosin stain). Only the serosa (s) appears intact. (*C*) Gross pathology at postmortem examination shows severe NEC. Arrows indicate severe sloughing of mucosa, submucosa, and muscularis mucosa. Only a thin layer of serosa is intact allowing the intestinal lumen to be seen. (*Adapted from* Epelman M, Daneman A, Navarro OM, et al. Necrotizing enterocolitis: review of state-of-the-art imaging findings with pathologic correlation. Radiographics 2007;27:285–305; with permission.)

DIFFERENTIAL DIAGNOSIS
IIP

It is more common for extremely premature infants with NEC to develop pneumoperitoneum than pneumatosis.[7] This population is also more vulnerable to IIP. Infants with IIP are generally more stable but they can develop peritonitis and sepsis syndrome mimicking NEC.[25,100,102] Generally, IIP presents during the first week of life and has been commonly associated with early indocin prophylaxis against intraventricular hemorrhage or patent ductus arteriosus (**Table 1**).[25] Pathologically IIP is a focal perforation without an inflammatory component. It is not associated with feeding and does not present as hemorrhagic ischemic necrosis.[25]

In contrast with the multifactorial pathogenesis of NEC, IIP usually develops suddenly without clinical evidence of intestinal inflammation.[25] The propensity for these focal lesions to occur in the watershed areas of terminal ileum or jejunum supports the theory of arterial occlusion with embolism.[25,126–128] Arterial rectae are end arteries that supply intestinal villi.[126–128] Persistence of right to left shunt through a patent foramen ovale or PDA during the early critical postnatal period presents a scenario for arterial embolism that potentially can create lesions similar to IIP, especially when these lesions occur near the antimesenteric border.[25]

Table 1
Comparison between IIP and NEC

Characteristics	IIP (n = 26)	NEC (n = 113)
Birth weight, mean ± SD (g)	828 ± 203	923 ± 202
Gestational age at birth, mean ± SD (wk)	25.9 ± 2.1	26.7 ± 2.0
Age at diagnosis (d)	6.7 ± 15.5	15.6 ± 9.1
Association with indomethacin (early, first dose on day 1)	Yes	No
Association with PDA	No	Yes
Predominant feature of pathophysiology	Circulatory	Inflammation
Mortality	42%	26%

Adapted from Sharma R, Hudak ML, Tepas JJ 3rd, et al. Prenatal or postnatal indomethacin exposure and neonatal gut injury associated with isolated intestinal perforation and necrotizing enterocolitis. J Perinatol 2010;30(12):786–93; with permission.

Sepsis

Sepsis can masquerade in a manner similar to NEC.[6] Many intestinal and systemic signs of sepsis also are characteristic of NEC. Specifically, ileus, hypotension, respiratory deterioration, thrombocytopenia, metabolic acidosis, left shift of neutrophils and neutropenia, and systemic inflammatory response syndrome (SIRS) also occur with septic shock unaccompanied by intestinal inflammation.[114] Although sepsis and SIRS are complications of NEC, it is important to exclude NEC as the underlying cause of sepsis. The following *two* findings, if present, favor the diagnosis of NEC:

- New-onset hyponatremia (<130 mEq/L) that cannot be explained by dilution or by treatment with diuretics (Generally, this finding appears early before significant clinical illness develops.)
- Hematochezia (blood in the stool, not occult blood) that may appear early in the disease process or later after resolution of ileus

The differential diagnosis also includes other causes of anatomic and functional intestinal obstruction (eg, malrotation, intestinal atresia, intussusceptions, aganglionosis); conditions that can result in intestinal ischemia (eg, volvulus, critical coarctation of the aorta, hypoplastic left heart syndrome); omphalitis; and milk protein intolerance.[8,9,105]

OUTCOMES AND COMPLICATIONS

The overall mortality rate in NEC is between 20% and 40% but varies with the severity and extent of gut necrosis.[129–131] Mortality is inversely related to PMA at birth.[6,15] Other complications of NEC include intestinal strictures, enterocutaneous fistula, intra-abdominal abscess, cholestasis, and short-bowel syndrome.[7,130,131] Intestinal and liver failure can also occur that requires transplantation. Strictures typically occur 3 to 8 weeks after the acute episode but can also present several months later.[97] Contrast enema is indicated if signs of subacute intestinal obstruction appear several weeks after the acute episode of NEC. The colon is the most common site for stricture development, but strictures can also occur in the ileum or jejunum.[97,98] Diffuse pneumatosis increases the risk for strictures.[97,98] Risks of all comorbidities of prematurity increase with NEC, including neurodevelopmental, motor, sensory, and cognitive problems.[129–134]

FUTURE DIRECTIONS
Prediction

The prediction of infants at an increased risk of NEC may be possible in the future through the use of methods that are currently available at a few research facilities. These methods use noninvasive indicators, such as profiling of the fecal micro-biome,[55] and the identification of the expression of inflammatory proteins from buccal epithelium using buccal swab collection.[135] The determination of oxidative stress by measuring concentrations of non–protein-bound iron, advanced oxidation protein products, and total hydroxides in cord blood has been reported to be useful in predicting which VP infants are at risk for NEC but requires additional validation.[136]

Predisposing Factors and Management Planning

Earlier noninvasive diagnosis of NEC through the use of abdominal sonography in infants with nonspecific clinical and radiographic signs and through the assessment of metabolic derangement may result in more timely and appropriate medical treatment and surgical intervention.[107,112] However, no studies have demonstrated improved clinical outcomes caused by facilitated diagnosis and management. Future trials comparing outcomes of peritoneal drainage with laparotomy should include distinguishing NEC from IIP.[100]

Perforation Versus NEC

Clinical studies suggest that the isolated perforation occurs when the intestinal mucosa has been weakened by processes, such as local ischemia-reperfusion or thromboembolism. Conversely, NEC involves both infectious and inflammatory mechanisms.[137] Designing strategies to prevent the occurrence of NEC and to improve outcomes of infants who develop NEC should consider these diagnoses as fundamentally different disease processes.

The focus of NEC research is shifting from concentrating on the distinct nature of this disease to understanding the unique characteristics of immune-naïve premature patients. Hence, investigative and interventional techniques aimed at ensuring a more appropriate and mature intestinal immune response should be tested as preventative strategies.

REFERENCES

1. Obladen M. Necrotizing enterocolitis –150 years of fruitless search of the cause. Neonatology 2009;96:203–10.
2. Mizrahi A, Barlow O, Berdon W, et al. Necrotizing enterocolitis in premature infants. J Pediatr 1965;66:697–705.
3. Touloukian RJ. Neonatal enterocolitis: an update on etiology, diagnosis, and treatment. Surg Clin North Am 1976;55:376–87.
4. Santulli TV, Schullinger JN, Heird WC, et al. Acute necrotizing enterocolitis in infancy: a review of 64 cases. Pediatrics 1975;55:376–87.
5. Bell MJ, Ternberg JL, Feigin RD, et al. Neonatal necrotizing enterocolitis. Therapeutic decisions based upon clinical staging. Ann Surg 1978;187(1):1–7.
6. Neu J, Walker WA. Necrotizing enterocolitis. N Engl J Med 2011;364(3):255–64.
7. Sharma R, Hudak ML, Tepas JJ 3rd, et al. Impact of gestational age on the clinical presentation and surgical outcome of necrotizing enterocolitis. J Perinatol 2006;26(6):342–7.

8. De La Torre CA, Miguel M, Martínez L, et al. The risk of necrotizing enterocolitis in newborns with congenital heart disease, a single institution-cohort study. Cir Pediatr 2010;23(2):103–6 [in Spanish].

9. Raboei EH. Necrotizing enterocolitis in full-term neonates: is it aganglionosis? Eur J Pediatr Surg 2009;19(2):101–4.

10. Snyder CL. Outcome analysis for gastroschisis. J Pediatr Surg 1999;34(8): 1253–6.

11. Thompson AM, Bizzarro MJ. Necrotizing enterocolitis in newborns: pathogenesis, prevention and management. Drugs 2008;68(9):1227–38.

12. Fanaroff AA, Stoll BJ, Wright LL, et al, NICHD Neonatal Research Network. Trends in neonatal morbidity and mortality for very low birth weight infants. Am J Obstet Gynecol 2007;196(2):147.e1–8.

13. Stoll BJ, Hansen NI, Bell EF. Neonatal outcomes of extremely preterm infants from the NICHD Neonatal Research Network. Pediatrics 2010;126(3):443–56.

14. Guillet R, Stoll BJ, Cotten CM, et al. Association of H2-blocker therapy and higher incidence of necrotizing enterocolitis in very low birth weight infants. Pediatrics 2006;117(2):e137–42.

15. Fitzgibbons SC, Ching Y, Yu D, et al. Mortality of necrotizing enterocolitis expressed by birth weight categories. J Pediatr Surg 2009;44(6):1072–5 [discussion: 1075–6].

16. EXPRESS group. Incidence of and risk factors for neonatal morbidity after active perinatal care: extremely preterm infants study in Sweden (EXPRESS). Acta Paediatr 2010;99(7):978–92.

17. Bajwa NM, Berner M, Worley S, et al, Swiss Neonatal Network. Population based age stratified morbidities of premature infants in Switzerland. Swiss Med Wkly 2011;141:w13212.

18. Yee WH, Soraisham AS, Shah VS, et al. Incidence and timing of presentation of necrotizing enterocolitis in preterm infants. Pediatrics 2012;129(2):e298–304.

19. Hunter CJ, Upperman JS, Ford HR, et al. Understanding the susceptibility of the premature infant to necrotizing enterocolitis (NEC). Pediatr Res 2008;63(2): 117–23.

20. Berrington JE, Hearn RI, Bythell M, et al. Deaths in preterm infants: changing pathology over 2 decades. J Pediatr 2012;160(1):49–53.e1.

21. Neu J, Mihatsch W. Recent developments in necrotizing enterocolitis. JPEN J Parenter Enteral Nutr 2012;36(Suppl 1):30S–5S.

22. Sharma R, Tepas JJ. Microecology, intestinal epithelial barrier and necrotizing enterocolitis. Pediatr Surg Int 2010;26:11–21.

23. Young CM, Kingma SD, Neu J. Ischemia-reperfusion and neonatal intestinal injury. J Pediatr 2011;158:e25–8.

24. Neu J. The myth of asphyxia and hypoxia-ischemia as primary causes of necrotizing enterocolitis. Biol Neonate 2005;87:97–8.

25. Sharma R, Hudak ML, Tepas JJ 3rd, et al. Prenatal or postnatal indomethacin exposure and neonatal gut injury associated with isolated intestinal perforation and necrotizing enterocolitis. J Perinatol 2010;30(12):786–93.

26. Nowicki PT, Caniano DA, Hammond S, et al. Endothelial nitric oxide synthase in human intestine resected for necrotizing enterocolitis. J Pediatr 2007;150(1): 40–5.

27. Nankervis CA, Giannone PJ, Reber KM. The neonatal intestinal vasculature: contributing factors to necrotizing enterocolitis. Semin Perinatol 2008;32:83–91.

28. Berseth CL. Gut motility and the pathogenesis of necrotizing enterocolitis. Clin Perinatol 1994;21(2):263–70.

29. Wu SF, Caplan M, Lin HC. Necrotizing enterocolitis: old problem with new hope. Pediatr Neonatol 2012;53(3):158–63.
30. Morowitz MJ, Poroyko V, Caplan M, et al. Redefining the role of intestinal microbes in the pathogenesis of necrotizing enterocolitis. Pediatrics 2010; 125(4):777–85.
31. Sharma R, Tepas JJ 3rd, Hudak ML, et al. Neonatal gut barrier and multiple organ failure: role of endotoxin and proinflammatory cytokines in sepsis and necrotizing enterocolitis. J Pediatr Surg 2007;42(3):454–61.
32. Ravindranath T, Yoshioka T, Goto M, et al. Endotoxemia following enteral refeeding in children. Clin Pediatr (Phila) 1997;36(9):523–8.
33. Kau A, Ahren PP, Griffin NW, et al. Human nutrition, the gut microbiome, and immune system: envisioning the future. Nature 2012;474(7351):327–36.
34. Liu Z, Li N, Neu J. Tight junctions, leaky intestines, and pediatric diseases. Acta Paediatr 2005;94(4):386–93.
35. Sharma R, Young C, Neu J. Molecular modulation of intestinal epithelial barrier: contribution of microbiota. J Biomed Biotechnol 2010;2010:305879.
36. Josephson CD, Wesolowski A, Bao G, et al. Do red cell transfusions increase the risk of necrotizing enterocolitis in premature infants? J Pediatr 2010;157(6): 972–978.e1–3.
37. Christensen RD, Lambert DK, Henry E, et al. Is "transfusion-associated necrotizing enterocolitis" an authentic pathogenic entity? Transfusion 2010;50(5): 1106–12.
38. Singh R, Visintainer PF, Frantz ID 3rd, et al. Association of necrotizing enterocolitis with anemia and packed red blood cell transfusions in preterm infants. J Perinatol 2011;31(3):176–82.
39. Paul DA, Mackley A, Novitsky A, et al. Increased odds of necrotizing enterocolitis after transfusion of red blood cells in premature infants. Pediatrics 2011; 127(4):635–41.
40. Blau J, Calo JM, Dozor D, et al. Transfusion-related acute gut injury: necrotizing enterocolitis in very low birth weight neonates after packed red blood cell transfusion. J Pediatr 2011;158(3):403–9.
41. dos Santos AM, Guinsburg R, de Almeida MF, et al, Brazilian Network on Neonatal Research. Red blood cell transfusions are independently associated with intra-hospital mortality in very low birth weight preterm infants. J Pediatr 2011;159(3):371–376.e1–3.
42. El-Dib M, Narang S, Lee E, et al. Red blood cell transfusion, feeding and necrotizing enterocolitis in preterm infants. J Perinatol 2011;31(3):183–7.
43. Afrazi A, Sodhi CP, Richardson W, et al. New insights into the pathogenesis and treatment of necrotizing enterocolitis: toll-like receptors and beyond. Pediatr Res 2011;69(3):183–8.
44. Neish AS. Microbes in gastrointestinal health and disease. Gastroenterology 2009;136(1):65–80.
45. Kawai T, Akira S. Toll-like receptors and their crosstalk with other innate receptors in infection and immunity. Immunity 2011;34(5):637–50.
46. Lin PW, Nasr TR, Stoll BJ. Necrotizing enterocolitis: recent scientific advances in pathophysiology and prevention. Semin Perinatol 2008;32(2):70–82.
47. Neu J, Chen M, Beierle E. Intestinal innate immunity: how does it relate to the pathogenesis of necrotizing enterocolitis. Semin Pediatr Surg 2005;14(3):137–44.
48. Nanthakumar N, Meng D, Goldstein AM, et al. The mechanism of excessive intestinal inflammation in necrotizing enterocolitis: an immature innate response. PLoS One 2011;6(3):e17776.

49. Ganguli K, Walker WA. Probiotics in the prevention of necrotizing enterocolitis. J Clin Gastroenterol 2011;45(Suppl):S133–8.
50. Lin PW, Myers LE, Ray L, et al. Lactobacillus rhamnosus blocks inflammatory signaling in vivo via reactive oxygen species generation. Free Radic Biol Med 2009;47(8):1205–11.
51. Alexander VN, Northrup V, Bizzarro MJ. Antibiotic exposure in the newborn intensive care unit and the risk of necrotizing enterocolitis. J Pediatr 2011; 159(3):392–7.
52. Cotten CM, Taylor S, Stoll B, et al. Prolonged duration of initial empirical antibiotic treatment is associated with increased rates of necrotizing enterocolitis and death for extremely low birth weight infants. Pediatrics 2009;123:58–66.
53. Bengmark S. Gut microbiota, immune development and function. Pharmacol Res 2012. pii: S1043–6618(12)00166-1. http://dx.doi.org/10.1016/j.phrs.2012.09.002.
54. Cilieborg MS, Boye M, Sangild PT. Bacterial colonization and gut development in preterm neonates. Early Hum Dev 2012;88(Suppl 1):S41–9 [Epub 2012 Jan 28].
55. Mai V, Young CM, Ukhanova M, et al. Fecal microbiota in premature infants prior to necrotizing enterocolitis. PLoS 2011;6(6):e20647.
56. Mohankumar K, Kaza N, Jagadeeswaran R, et al. Gut mucosal injury in neonates is marked by macrophage infiltration in contrast to pleomorphic infiltrates in adult: evidence from an animal model. Am J Physiol Gastrointest Liver Physiol 2012;303(1):G93–102.
57. Nanthakumar NN, Young C, Ko JS, et al. Glucocorticoid responsiveness in developing human intestine: possible role in prevention of necrotizing enterocolitis. Am J Physiol Gastrointest Liver Physiol 2005;288(1):G85–92.
58. Desfrere L, de Oliveira I, Goffinet F, et al. Increased incidence of necrotizing enterocolitis in premature infants born to HIV-positive mothers. AIDS 2005; 19(14):1487–93.
59. Cunningham SC, Fakhry K, Bass BL, et al. Neutropenic enterocolitis in adults: case series and review of the literature. Dig Dis Sci 2005;50(2):215–20.
60. Choi JH, Lee JM, Shin WS, et al. Necrotizing enterocolitis: experience of 27 cases from a single Korean institution. Int J Hematol 2000;72(3):358–61.
61. Downard CD, Grant SN, Matheson PJ, et al. Altered intestinal microcirculation is the critical event in the development of necrotizing enterocolitis. J Pediatr Surg 2011;46(6):1023–8.
62. Kim M, Christley S, Alverdy JC, et al. Immature oxidative stress management as a unifying principle in the pathogenesis of necrotizing enterocolitis: insights from an agent-based model. Surg Infect (Larchmt) 2012;13(1):18–32 [Epub 2012 Jan 4].
63. Chokshi NK, Guner YS, Hunter CJ, et al. The role of nitric oxide in intestinal epithelial injury and restitution in neonatal necrotizing enterocolitis [review]. Semin Perinatol 2008;32(2):92–9.
64. Li N, Quidgley MC, Kobeissy FH, et al. Microbial cell components induced tolerance to flagellin-stimulated inflammation through Toll-like receptor pathways in intestinal epithelial cells. Cytokine 2012;60(3):806–11 [PMID: 22944462].
65. Smith B, Bodé S, Skov TH, et al. Investigation of the early intestinal microflora in premature infants with/without necrotizing enterocolitis using two different methods. Pediatr Res 2012;71(1):115–20.
66. Peter CS, Feuerhahn M, Bohnhorst B, et al. Necrotising enterocolitis: is there a relationship to specific pathogens? Eur J Pediatr 1999;158:67–70.

67. Powell J, Bureau MA, Pare C, et al. Necrotizing enterocolitis. Epidemic following an outbreak of Enterobacter cloacae type 3305573 in a neonatal intensive care unit. Am J Dis Child 1980;134:1152–4.
68. Mollitt DL, Tepas JJ 3rd, Talbert JL. The microbiology of neonatal peritonitis. Arch Surg 1988;123:176–9.
69. Howard FM, Flynn DM, Bradley JM, et al. Outbreak of necrotising enterocolitis caused by Clostridium butyricum. Lancet 1977;2:1099–102.
70. Van Acker J, de Smet F, Muyldermans G, et al. Outbreak of necrotizing enterocolitis associated with Enterobacter sakazakii in powdered milk formula. J Clin Microbiol 2001;39:293–7.
71. Smith B, Bodé S, Petersen BL, et al. Community analysis of bacteria colonizing intestinal tissue of neonates with necrotizing enterocolitis. BMC Microbiol 2011; 11:73. http://dx.doi.org/10.1186/1471-2180-11-73.
72. Tzialla C, Civardi E, Borghesi A, et al. Emerging viral infections in neonatal intensive care unit. J Matern Fetal Neonatal Med 2011;24(Suppl 1):156–8 [Epub 2011 Aug 31].
73. Sharma R, Hudak ML, Premachandra BR, et al. Clinical manifestations of rotavirus infection in the neonatal intensive care unit. Pediatr Infect Dis J 2002; 21(12):1099–105.
74. Stuart RL, Tan K, Mahar JE, et al. An outbreak of necrotizing enterocolitis associated with norovirus genotype GII.3. Pediatr Infect Dis J 2010;29(7):644–7.
75. Sharma R, Garrison RD, Tepas JJ 3rd, et al. Rotavirus-associated necrotizing enterocolitis: an insight into a potentially preventable disease? J Pediatr Surg 2004;39(3):453–7.
76. Birenbaum E, Handsher R, Kuint J, et al. Echovirus type 22 outbreak associated with gastro-intestinal disease in a neonatal intensive care unit. Am J Perinatol 1997;14:469–73.
77. Chany C, Moscovici O, Lebon P, et al. Association of coronavirus infection with neonatal necrotizing enterocolitis. Pediatrics 1982;69:209–14.
78. Bagci S, Eis-Hübinger AM, Franz AR, et al. Detection of astrovirus in premature infants with necrotizing enterocolitis. Pediatr Infect Dis J 2008;27(4): 347–50.
79. Lodha A, de Silva N, Petric M, et al. Human torovirus: a new virus associated with neonatal necrotizing enterocolitis. Acta Paediatr 2005;94:1085–8.
80. Karlowicz MG. Risk factors associated with fungal peritonitis in very low birth weight neonates with severe necrotizing enterocolitis: a case-control study. Pediatr Infect Dis J 1993;12:574–7.
81. Boccia D, Stolfi I, Lana S, et al. Nosocomial necrotizing outbreaks: epidemiology and control measures. Eur J Pediatr 2001;160:385–91.
82. Lemyre B, Xiu W, Bouali NR, et al. A decrease in the number of cases of necrotizing enterocolitis associated with the enhancement of infection prevention and control measures during a Staphylococcus aureus outbreak in a neonatal intensive care unit. Infect Control Hosp Epidemiol 2012;33(1):29–33.
83. Faustini A, Forastiere F, Giorgi-Rossi P, et al. An epidemic of gastroenteritis and mild necrotizing enterocolitis in two neonatal units of a university hospital in Rome, Italy. Epidemiol Infect 2004;132(3):455–65.
84. Turcios-Ruiz RM, Axelrod P, St John K, et al. Outbreak of necrotizing enterocolitis caused by norovirus in a neonatal intensive care unit. J Pediatr 2008;153(3): 339–44.
85. Chappé C, Minjolle S, Dabadie A, et al. Astrovirus and digestive disorders in neonatal units. Acta Paediatr 2012;101(5):e208–12.

86. Moscovici O, Chany C, Lebon P, et al. Association of coronavirus infection with hemorrhagic enterocolitis in newborn infants. C R Seances Acad Sci D 1980; 290(13):869–72 [in French].
87. Bagci S, Eis-Hübinger AM, Yassin AF, et al. Clinical characteristics of viral intestinal infection in preterm and term neonates. Eur J Clin Microbiol Infect Dis 2010; 29(9):1079–84.
88. Ball JM, Tian P, Zeng CQ, et al. Age-dependent diarrhea induced by rotavirus nonstructural glycoprotein. Science 1996;272:101–4.
89. Guttman JA, Finlay BB. Tight junctions as targets of infectious agents. Biochim Biophys Acta 2009;1788(4):832–41.
90. Morris AP, Estes MK. Microbes and microbial toxins: paradigms for microbial-mucosal interactions. VIII. Pathological consequences of rotavirus infection and its enterotoxin. Am J Physiol Gastrointest Liver Physiol 2001;281(2):G303–10.
91. Schroeder ME, Hosteller HA, Schroeder F, et al. Elucidation of the rotavirus NSP4-caveolin-1 and-cholesterol interactions using synthetic peptides. J Amino acids 2012;2012:575180. http://dx.doi.org/10.1155/2012/575180.
92. Neish AS. The gut microflora and intestinal epithelial cells: a continuing dialogue. Microbes infect 2002;4:309–17.
93. Cilieborg MS, Boye M, Mølbak L, et al. Preterm birth and necrotizing enterocolitis alter gut colonization in pigs. Pediatr Res 2011;69(1):10–6.
94. Kliegman RM, Hack M, Jones P, et al. Epidemiological study of necrotizing enterocolitis among low birth weight infants. J Pediatr 1982;100:440–4.
95. Kanto WP Jr, Hunter JE, Stoll BJ. Recognition and medical management of necrotizing enterocolitis. Clin Perinatol 1994;21(2):335–46.
96. Gephart SM, McGrath JM, Effken JA, et al. Necrotizing enterocolitis risk: state of the science. Adv Neonatal Care 2012;12(2):77–87.
97. Sharma R, Tepas JJ 3rd, Hudak ML, et al. Portal venous gas and surgical outcome of neonatal necrotizing enterocolitis. J Pediatr Surg 2005;40(2):371–6.
98. Faix RG, Nelson M. Neonatal enterocolitis: progress, problems, and prospects. In: David TJ, editor. Recent advances in Paediatrics, vol. 16. Edinburgh: Churchill Livingstone; 1998. p. 359–407.
99. Abramo TJ, Evans JS, Kokomoor FW, et al. Occult blood in stools and necrotizing enterocolitis. Am J Dis Child 1988;142:451–2.
100. Sharma R, Tepas JJ 3rd, Mollitt DL, et al. Surgical management of bowel perforations and outcome in very low-birth-weight infants (≤1,200 g). J Pediatr Surg 2004;39(2):190–4.
101. Cole CR, Hansen NI, Higgins RD, et al, Eunice Kennedy Shriver National Institute of Child Health and Human Development's Neonatal Research Network. Bloodstream infections in very low birth weight infants with intestinal failure. J Pediatr 2012;160(1):54–59.e2.
102. Sharma R, Tepas JJ 3rd, Hudak ML, et al. Neonatal gut injury and infection rate: impact of surgical debridement on outcome. Pediatr Surg Int 2005;21(12):977–82.
103. Stringer MD, Brereton RJ, Drake DP, et al. Recurrent necrotizing enterocolitis. J Pediatr Surg 1993;28(8):979–81.
104. Srinivasan P, Brandler M, D'Souza A, et al. Allergic enterocolitis presenting as recurrent necrotizing enterocolitis in preterm neonates. J Perinatol 2010;30(6):431–3.
105. Coviello C, Rodriquez DC, Cecchi S, et al. Different clinical manifestation of cow's milk allergy in two preterm twins newborns. J Matern Fetal Neonatal Med 2012;25(Suppl 1):132–3.
106. Morrison SC, Jacobson JM. The radiology of necrotizing enterocolitis. Clin Perinatol 1994;21(2):347–63.

107. Epelman M, Daneman A, Navarro OM, et al. Necrotizing enterocolitis: review of state-of-the-art imaging findings with pathologic correlation. Radiographics 2007;27:285–305.
108. Faingold R, Daneman A, Tomlinson G, et al. Necrotizing enterocolitis: assessment of bowel viability with color Doppler US. Radiology 2005;235(2):587–94.
109. Kanto WP Jr, Wilson R, Ricketts RR. Management and outcome of necrotizing enterocolitis. Clin Pediatr (Phila) 1985;24(2):79–82.
110. Walsh MC, Kliegman RM. Necrotizing enterocolitis: treatment based on staging criteria. Pediatr Clin North Am 1986;33(1):179–201.
111. Neu J. Neonatal necrotizing enterocolitis: an update. Acta Paediatr Suppl 2005; 94(449):100–5.
112. Tepas JJ 3rd, Leaphart CL, Plumley D, et al. Trajectory of metabolic derangement in infants with necrotizing enterocolitis should drive timing and technique of surgical intervention. J Am Coll Surg 2010;210:847–52.
113. Musemeche CA, Kosloske AM, Ricketts RR. Enterostomy in necrotizing enterocolitis: an analysis of techniques and timing of closure. J Pediatr Surg 1987; 22(6):479–83.
114. Tepas JJ 3rd, Sharma R, Leaphart CL, et al. Timing of surgical intervention in necrotizing enterocolitis can be determined by trajectory of metabolic derangement. J Pediatr Surg 2010;45(2):310–3 [discussion: 313–4].
115. Ein SH, Shandling B, Wesson D, et al. A 13-year experience with peritoneal drainage under local anesthesia for necrotizing enterocolitis perforation. J Pediatr Surg 1990;25:1034–6.
116. Rao SC, Basani L, Simmer K, et al. Peritoneal drainage versus laparotomy as initial surgical treatment for perforated necrotizing enterocolitis or spontaneous intestinal perforation in preterm low birth weight infants. Cochrane Database Syst Rev 2011;(6):CD006182.
117. Rees CM, Eaton S, Kiely EM, et al. Peritoneal drainage or laparotomy for neonatal bowel perforation? A randomized controlled trial. Ann Surg 2008; 248:44–51.
118. Moss RL, Dimmit RA, Barnhart DC, et al. Laparotomy versus peritoneal drainage for necrotizing enterocolitis. N Engl J Med 2006;354:2225–34.
119. Pierro A, Eaton S, Rees CM, et al. Is there a benefit of peritoneal drainage for necrotizing enterocolitis in newborn infants? J Pediatr Surg 2010;45:2117–8.
120. Blakely ML, Tyson JE, Lally KP, et al. Laparotomy versus peritoneal drainage for necrotizing enterocolitis or isolated intestinal perforation in extremely low birth weight infants: outcomes through 18 months adjusted age. Pediatrics 2006; 117(4):e680–7.
121. Sola JE, Tepas JJ 3rd, Koniaris LG. Peritoneal drainage versus laparotomy for necrotizing enterocolitis and intestinal perforation: a meta-analysis. J Surg Res 2010;161(1):95–100.
122. Tepas JJ 3rd, Sharma R, Hudak ML, et al. Coming full circle: an evidence-based definition of the timing and type of surgical management of very low-birth-weight (<1000 g) infants with signs of acute intestinal perforation. J Pediatr Surg 2006; 41(2):418–22.
123. Kosloske AM. Indications for operation in necrotizing enterocolitis revisited. J Pediatr Surg 1994;29(5):663–6.
124. Ballance WA, Dahms BB, Shenker N, et al. Pathology of necrotizing enterocolitis: a ten year experience. J Pediatr 1990;117:S6–13.
125. Gould SJ. The pathology of necrotizing enterocolitis. Semin Neonatol 1997;4: 239–44.

126. Jacobs JE, Birnbaum BA, Maglinte DD. Vascular disorders of the small intestine. In: Herlinger H, Maglinte DD, Birnbaum BA, editors. Clinical imaging of the small intestine. 2nd edition. New York: Springer-Verlag; 1999. p. 439–65.

127. Nankervis CA, Reber KM, Nowicki PT. Age-dependent changes in the postnatal intestinal microcirculation. Microcirculation 2001;8(6):377–87.

128. Nowicki PT, Miller CE, Edwards RC. Effects of hypoxia and ischemia on autoregulation in postnatal intestine. Am J Physiol 1991;261:G152–7.

129. Sankaran K, Puckett B, Lee DS, et al, Canadian Neonatal Network. Variations in incidence of necrotizing enterocolitis in Canadian neonatal intensive care units. J Pediatr Gastroenterol Nutr 2004;39(4):366–72.

130. Abdullah F, Zhang Y, Camp M, et al. Necrotizing enterocolitis in 20,822 infants: analysis of medical and surgical treatments. Clin Pediatr (Phila) 2010;49(2): 166–71.

131. Guner YS, Friedlich P, Wee CP, et al. State-based analysis of necrotizing enterocolitis outcomes. J Surg Res 2009;157(1):21–9.

132. Martin CR, Dammann O, Allred EN, et al. Neurodevelopment of extremely preterm infants who had necrotizing enterocolitis with or without late bacteremia. J Pediatr 2010;157(5):751–756.e1.

133. Shah DK, Doyle LW, Anderson PJ, et al. Adverse neurodevelopment in preterm infants with postnatal sepsis or necrotizing enterocolitis is mediated by white matter abnormalities on magnetic resonance imaging at term. J Pediatr 2008; 153(2):170–5, 175.e1 [Epub 2008 Apr 3].

134. Pike K, Brocklehurst P, Jones D, et al. Outcomes at 7 years for babies who developed neonatal necrotising enterocolitis: the ORACLE Children Study. Arch Dis Child Fetal Neonatal Ed 2012;97(5):F318–22.

135. Warner BB, Ryan AL, Seeger K, et al. Ontogeny of salivary epidermal growth factor and necrotizing enterocolitis. J Pediatr 2007;150(4):358–63.

136. Perrone S, Tataranno ML, Negro S, et al. May oxidative stress biomarkers in cord blood predict the occurrence of necrotizing enterocolitis in preterm infants? J Matern Fetal Neonatal Med 2012;25(Suppl 1):128–31.

137. Chan KY, Leung FW, Lam HS, et al. Immunoregulatory protein profiles of necrotizing enterocolitis versus spontaneous intestinal perforation in preterm infants. PLoS One 2012;7(5):e36977.

Short Bowel Syndrome in the NICU

Sachin C. Amin, MD[a], Cleo Pappas, MLIS[b], Hari Iyengar, MD[a],
Akhil Maheshwari, MD[a,c],*

KEYWORDS

- Short gut • Intestinal adaptation • Intestinal rehabilitation • Short bowel syndrome
- Necrotizing enterocolitis • Malabsorption • Small bowel transplant
- Bowel conservation

KEY POINTS

- In neonatal intensive care units, the most common cause of intestinal failure is surgical short bowel syndrome, which is defined as a need for prolonged parenteral nutrition following bowel resection, usually for more than 3 months.
- The clinical course of short bowel syndrome patients can be described in the 3 following clinical stages: acute, recovery, and maintenance.
- A cohesive, multidisciplinary approach can allow most infants with SBS to transition to full enteral feeds and achieve normal growth and development.

DEFINITIONS: INTESTINAL FAILURE AND SHORT BOWEL SYNDROME

Intestinal failure is defined as a significant reduction in the functional gut mass below a critical threshold necessary to maintain growth, hydration, and/or electrolyte balance.[1,2] Intestinal failure can occur because of surgical resection of bowel, congenital anomalies, or functional/motility disorders. In neonatal intensive care units (NICUs), the most common cause of intestinal failure is the surgical short bowel syndrome (SBS), which is defined as a need for prolonged parenteral nutrition following bowel resection, usually for more than 3 months.[3]

Conflicts of Interest: The authors disclose no conflicts.
Funding: National Institutes of Health award R01HD059142 (to A.M.).
[a] Department of Pediatrics, Division of Neonatology, Center for Neonatal and Pediatric Gastrointestinal Disease, University of Illinois at Chicago, 840 South Wood Street, CSB 1257, Chicago, IL 60612, USA; [b] Department of Medical Education, Library of Health Sciences, University of Illinois at Chicago, 1750 West Polk Street, Chicago, IL 60612, USA; [c] Division of Neonatology, Department of Pharmacology, Center for Neonatal and Pediatric Gastrointestinal Disease, University of Illinois at Chicago, 840 South Wood Street, CSB 1257, Chicago, IL 60612, USA
* Corresponding author. Department of Pediatrics, Division of Neonatology, Center for Neonatal and Pediatric Gastrointestinal Disease, University of Illinois at Chicago, 840 South Wood Street, CSB 1257, Chicago, IL 60612.
E-mail address: akhil1@uic.edu

EPIDEMIOLOGY OF SBS IN NEONATES AND YOUNG INFANTS

Surgical SBS was recorded in 0.7% (89/12,316) of very low birth weight infants born during the period 2002 to 2005 at the National Institute of Child Health and Development neonatal research network centers.[4] The frequency of SBS increased in an inverse relationship with birth weight; the incidence of SBS in infants weighing 401 to 1000 g was 1.1% (61/5657), nearly twice that in infants with a birth weight of 1001 to 1500 g (28/6659; 0.4%).[4] In Canada, data from a large tertiary NICU show an overall incidence of SBS as 22.1 per 1000 admissions, and 24.5 per 100,000 live births.[5] The incidence was higher in infants born at less than 37 weeks' gestation (353.7 per 100,000 live births) than in full-term infants (3.5/100,000 live births). The SBS rate of case fatality was 37.5%.[5] Similarly, in a study from 7 tertiary neonatal units in Italy, intestinal failure was seen in 0.1% (26/30,353) of all live births and 0.5% (26/5088) among those admitted to the NICU.[6]

Attempts to estimate the incidence and prevalence of SBS have been constrained by the rarity of the condition, variation in nomenclature, difficulty in providing a clear definition of the study population at tertiary institutions because of complex referral patterns, and paucity of follow-up data.[3,5] Population-based studies are sparse. Although the need for home parenteral nutrition has been used as a surrogate for SBS in some studies, this approach has important limitations; some patients may require parenteral nutrition because of a diagnosis other than SBS, such as malignancy, whereas some infants with SBS who may have been weaned off parenteral nutrition before discharge from the hospital may not be included.

CAUSE OF SBS IN NEONATES AND YOUNG INFANTS

Necrotizing enterocolitis (NEC) is the most common cause of SBS (35%) in neonates, followed by intestinal atresia (25%), gastroschisis (18%), malrotation with volvulus (14%), followed by less common conditions, such as Hirschsprung disease with proximal extension of aganglionosis into the small bowel (2%) (**Fig. 1**).[2] In another study, infants with SBS who eventually required intestinal transplantation had the following primary diagnoses: gastroschisis (25%), intestinal volvulus (24%), NEC (12%), intestinal pseudo-obstruction (10%), jejunoileal atresia (9%), Hirschsprungs disease (7%), and other conditions (13%).[7] In very low birth weight infants, NEC remains the predominant cause of SBS. In the National Institute of Child Health and Development cohort, 96% of cases of SBS were due to NEC. Congenital defects (gastroschisis, intestinal atresia) accounted for 2% and volvulus accounted for the remaining 2%.[4]

Duro and colleagues[8] enrolled 473 patients with a diagnosis of NEC. Among the 129 patients who required surgery, 54 (42%) developed SBS, which was significantly more

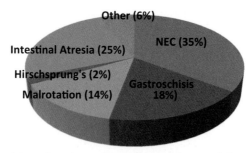
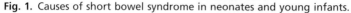

Fig. 1. Causes of short bowel syndrome in neonates and young infants.

common than in the control group (6/265; 2%; odds ratio [OR] 31.1, 95% confidence interval, 12.9–75.1, $P<.001$). Multivariate analysis showed that SBS was associated with variables characteristic of severe NEC: birth weight less than 750 g (OR = 9.09, $P<.001$), antibiotic use (OR = 16.61, P = .022), ventilator use on day of diagnosis (OR = 6.16, P = .009), exposure to enteral feeding before the diagnosis of NEC (OR = 4.05, P = .048), and percentage of small bowel resected (OR = 1.85 per 10% point greater resection, P = .031).

Besides NEC, gastroschisis is now emerging as a common cause of pediatric SBS leading to intestinal transplantation.[7,9] The incidence of gastroschisis is increasing and has been estimated in recent studies to be as high as 5 per 10,000 live births.[10,11] In gastroschisis, the fetal bowel eviscerates through a narrow abdominal wall defect and in the absence of a covering membrane, is exposed to the amniotic fluid. Patients with gastroschisis can develop SBS because of associated jejunoileal atresia, malrotation, and consequent midgut volvulus, and occasionally, because of refractory intestinal failure.[7]

Intestinal atresia, seen in approximately 1 in 5000 newborns, is another important cause of SBS in the NICU.[2] Although most patients with jejunoileal atresia have an isolated atretic segment that can be treated by a simple resection and end-to-end anastomosis, some infants with severe disruption develop SBS. When a major blood vessel such as the superior mesenteric artery is occluded in utero, large parts of bowel can become atretic. In about 10% of all cases of intestinal atresia, these disrupted bowel loops lack a dorsal mesentery and can assume a spiral configuration resembling an "apple peel."[12] In a series of 15 infants,[13] apple-peel intestinal atresia was associated with increased postoperative morbidity and mortality. Two of these 15 infants had SBS at 24 months. Infants with multiple intestinal atresias ("sausage-string"-type defect) are also at risk of SBS.[14,15]

SBS can occur in infants with Hirschsprung disease, particularly in those at the severe end of the spectrum with proximal extension of aganglionosis into the small intestine.[16] Some infants with Hirschsprung disease can develop intestinal failure and SBS after severe enterocolitis and associated tissue necrosis.[17]

CLINICAL PRESENTATION OF INFANTS WITH SBS

The clinical course of SBS patients can be described in the 3 following clinical stages:

Stage I (acute phase): After recovery from postoperative ileus, most patients go into an acute phase starting at about 1 week after surgery and lasting for up to 3 weeks.[18,19] This phase is characterized by large fluid and electrolyte losses in ostomy effluent/stool, requiring intravenous fluids and parenteral nutrition. Medical management is aimed at maintenance of the fluid and electrolyte balance. Depending on the extent of intestinal resection, the acute phase is generally associated with gastric hypersecretion. Treatment with H2 blockers or proton pump inhibitors may become necessary during this stage.

Stage II (recovery phase): The second stage starts after a few weeks and continues for several months.[18,19] This phase is characterized by gradual improvement in diarrhea and ostomy output. The dependence on parenteral nutrition is related to the degree of initial intestinal loss, condition of the remaining bowel at the time of the surgery, and compensatory histoarchitectural changes in the residual gut mucosa. Clinical management during this stage involves cautious initiation of enteral nutrition and gradual weaning of parenteral nutrition.

Stage III (maintenance phase): The third stage indicates successful intestinal adaptation.[18,19] In this stage, enteral nutrition is tolerated and parenteral nutrition can be discontinued. Oral feedings can often be started at this stage. The time required to reach this stage is variable depending on the infant's clinical course and complications.

The term "intestinal adaptation" is used in the clinical setting to indicate the recovery of intestinal function after intestinal resection.[20] Intestinal adaptation starts as early as 48 hours after surgery and may continue for up to 18 months. This intestinal adaptation contrasts with another frequently used term, "intestinal rehabilitation," which is used to describe the compensatory changes in the mucosal histoarchitecture and function in the residual bowel, which can increase the absorptive surface area and restore the capacity of the remaining intestine to absorb fluid, electrolytes, and nutrients in adequate amounts to meet the growth and maintenance requirements of the body. Typical rehabilitative changes in the mucosa include axial lengthening of the villi, deepening of the crypts, increased enterocyte proliferation, which increases enterocyte counts per villus, and enhanced enterocyte function with increased nutrient uptake.[21]

In SBS, the clinical presentation and outcome depend on the length and health of the remaining bowel, age of the patient, gastrointestinal regions that were resected and are now missing, presence of ileocecal valve, and other comorbidities.[3,22] The length of the remaining intestine is arguably the most important determinant of clinical outcome in SBS. Age is another important factor, and the potential for intestinal growth is much better in infants than in adults. Intestinal length increases from 142 $\pm$ 22 cm at 19 to 27 weeks of gestation to 217 $\pm$ 24 cm at 27 to 35 weeks, and to 304 $\pm$ 44 cm at term (range, 176–305 cm).[23,24] Small bowel growth peaks at 25 to 35 weeks' gestation and doubles in length during the last 15 weeks of pregnancy. After birth, the intestine continues to grow at a rapid rate until the crown-heel length reaches 60 cm and then at a slightly slower pace until the mature intestinal length of 600 to 700 cm is reached about when the somatic height approaches 100 to 140 cm.[25]

Studies show that in the absence of surgical bowel lengthening and tapering procedures, an infant with about 35 cm of residual small bowel has a 50% probability of being weaned from parenteral nutrition.[26] In other series, the likelihood of developing SBS following bowel resection was greater when the residual intestinal length was less than 25% of the predicted length for a given gestational age.[5] In another study, Wilmore[27] reported that an infant with SBS was more likely to survive if the small intestinal length was at least 15 cm in the presence of an intact ileocecal valve, or 40 cm in the absence of the ileocecal valve. Consistent with these observations, Spencer and colleagues[22] noted that a bowel length of less than 10% of expected length was associated with increased mortality (relative risk, 5.74).[22] In this series, 88% (52/59) of all infants retaining $\geq$10% of their expected normal small intestinal length survived, compared with only 21% (4/19) of those with less than 10% of expected length. With a given intestinal length, outcomes may also vary depending on the quality of the remaining bowel, region of the gastrointestinal tract, and the gestational age of the patient. There are reports of some infants who were weaned successfully from parenteral nutrition with as little as 10 cm residual intestinal length.[26] Generally, premature infants have a greater capacity for intestinal growth and adaptation as compared with full-term newborns.[26]

In a given patient, the clinical features of SBS can usually be predicted based on the gastrointestinal regions that were lost to surgical resection (**Fig. 2**).[3,22] Jejunal resection is usually tolerated relatively well because the ileal mucosa can adapt to compensate for the lost absorptive surface area. The loss of jejunum can affect intestinal motility in the postsurgical period and has also been associated with increased gastric emptying. Decreased production of cholecystokinin, secretin, vasoactive intestinal peptide, and serotonin in these patients can lead to gastrin hypersecretion, causing increased basal and peak acid output.

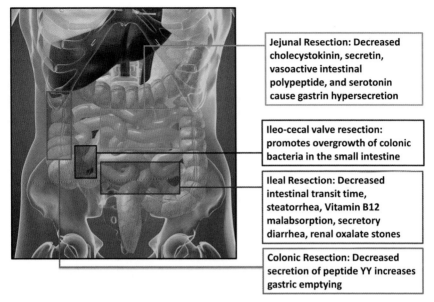

Jejunal Resection: Decreased cholecystokinin, secretin, vasoactive intestinal polypeptide, and serotonin cause gastrin hypersecretion

Ileo-cecal valve resection: promotes overgrowth of colonic bacteria in the small intestine

Ileal Resection: Decreased intestinal transit time, steatorrhea, Vitamin B12 malabsorption, secretory diarrhea, renal oxalate stones

Colonic Resection: Decreased secretion of peptide YY increases gastric emptying

Fig. 2. Clinical features of short bowel syndrome can be predicted based on the gastrointestinal region(s) that were lost to surgical resection and resulting physiologic changes.

Compared to patients with jejunal resection, ileal resection is more often associated with symptoms because the capacity of jejunum to compensate for the lost ileum is limited.[28] Ileal resection is frequently associated with impaired absorption of fluid and electrolytes, bile acids, and vitamin B_{12}. Decreased bile acid reabsorption can result in a reduced bile acid pool, leading to impaired micelle formation, fat malabsorption, and steatorrhea. In these patients, removal of the ileocecal valve is another negative predictor of clinical outcome. The ileocecal valve is presumed to play an important role in the regulation of gut bacterial flora by preventing retrograde migration and overgrowth of colonic bacteria, which thrive in areas of intestinal dilatation, and impaired motility. Colonic bacteria can deconjugate unabsorbed bile acids, which, in turn, can stimulate the gut epithelium and cause secretory diarrhea.

Colonic resection can increase the risk of fluid and electrolyte depletion and dehydration. Colonic resection can also increase gastric emptying and reduce intestinal transit time because of decreased secretion of peptide YY, glucagon-like peptide 1 (GLP-1), and neurotensin, which are important negative regulators of gut motility.[29] Overall, preservation of colon is associated with better outcomes in the case of SBS patients.

Several studies have shown that plasma levels of citrulline, a nonstructural amino acid synthesized in the intestinal mucosa, is a useful marker for estimating the total functional intestinal mass.[30,31] Serum citrulline concentrations correlate with the length of the remaining small intestinal bowel in patients with SBS[30] and also with the ability of the patient to be weaned from parenteral nutrition. Rhoads and colleagues[32] showed that serum citrulline levels show a linear correlation with the percentage of enteral calories and bowel length. A serum citrulline level ≥ 19 μmol/L was associated with enteral tolerance and was predictive of weaning from parenteral nutrition. In another study, Fitzgibbons and colleagues[33] showed that patients with plasma levels of citrulline less than 12 μmol/L could not be weaned off parenteral nutrition.

SBS is associated with increased rates of morbidity and mortality. Infants with SBS are at risk of sepsis, prolonged hospitalization, growth delay, and motor developmental delay.[34] Infants with SBS have a 3-fold increase in mortality than in controls, who had the same underlying condition but no SBS (37.5% [15/40] vs 13/3% [18/135]). Infants with SBS have disease-specific rates of mortality that are 5 times higher than those without SBS—20.2 versus 3.8 per 100 person-years.[3,5] SBS-related mortality tends to be highest in the early postoperative period and then decreases until 200 to 350 days after surgery, when a second peak in mortality is associated with the onset of end-stage liver disease.[35]

COMPLICATIONS OF SBS
Gastric Acid Hypersecretion

Gastric acid hypersecretion is seen in approximately 50% of all patients with SBS.[36,37] Proximal intestinal resection may be more likely to increase acid output than distal resection. Increased gastric output in SBS can predispose to acid-peptic injury, exacerbate fluid and electrolyte losses, impair intraluminal digestion, and cause malabsorption by causing inactivation of pancreatic exocrine enzymes, precipitation of bile salts (and ineffective micelle formation), and physical damage to the small bowel mucosa.

In SBS, increased circulating levels of gastrin are widely believed to be the primary reason for acid hypersecretion. In 1 study, arterial levels of gastrin were higher than in mesenteric veins draining the distal small bowel, indicating that intestine is a site for gastrin metabolism and that increased gastrin concentrations in patients with SBS may be due to disruption of this process. Another possibility is the loss of an inhibitor that is normally produced in the intestine and blocks gastrin action; secretin, gastrointestinal inhibitory polypeptide, cholecystokinin, and somatostatin have been proposed as candidates.[36]

Bacterial Overgrowth

Bacterial overgrowth is seen in up to 60% of all patients with SBS.[2] Expansion of the bacterial flora can result in deconjugation of bile acids, competition for metabolites, consumption of enteral nutrients and vitamins, accumulation of toxic metabolites such as D-lactate, and bacterial translocation producing bloodstream infections.[38] Clinical signs of bacterial overgrowth include abdominal pain, anorexia, vomiting, diarrhea, cramps, and metabolic acidosis from accumulation of D-lactic acid.

D-Lactic Acidosis

D-Lactic acidosis is a classic complication of bacterial overgrowth.[2,39] Intestinal bacteria produce both L-lactate and D-lactate, of which only L-lactate is metabolized. D-lactate can accumulate to toxic levels, sometimes causing neurologic problems ranging from disorientation to coma. D-Lactic acidosis is characterized by increased anion gap acidosis with normal levels of L-lactate. Strategies to prevent D-lactic acidosis include the administration of antibiotics to control bacterial overgrowth and reducing carbohydrate intake in patients with partial enteral nutrition.

Translocation of Enteric Bacteria

Translocation of enteric bacteria to the bloodstream is an important complication of SBS with bacterial overgrowth. In animal models, aerobic bacteria translocate more readily than anaerobic bacteria.[38,40] Treatment of bacterial overgrowth is empiric: broad spectrum antibiotics effective against enteric bacteria are administered for

7 to 14 days; followed by "rest" for 14 to 21 days; and then the cycle is repeated. Because many patients with SBS are dependent on parenteral nutrition and have central lines that can provide a nidus for infection, bacterial translocation in these patients increases the risk of central line–associated bloodstream infections. The frequency of catheter-related infections in children with SBS has been estimated as 11 to 26 infections per 1000 catheter-days.[41,42] Catheter-associated sepsis may require the removal of the line and with repeated infections, eventually leading to the loss of central venous access sites, accelerated liver failure, and increased mortality. Clinical signs of central line infections include fever, irritability, and ileus. Catheter-related infections can be minimized by the use of strict aseptic techniques during insertion, maintenance of sterile occlusive dressings, close surveillance for signs of infection, and the use of antibiotic-impregnated catheters and antibiotic and/or ethanol locks. In a recent study, Jones and colleagues[41] reported successful use of 70% (v/v) ethanol locks in 23 patients with SBS. Ethanol locks were well-tolerated with no reported adverse effects. Rates of infection decreased from 9.9 per 1000 catheter-days in historical controls to 2.2 per 1000 catheter-days during the period when ethanol locks were used.

Intestinal Failure-Associated Liver Disease

Intestinal failure-associated liver disease develops in 40% to 60% of infants who require long-term parenteral nutrition for intestinal failure. The clinical spectrum includes hepatic steatosis, cholestasis, cholelithiasis, and hepatic fibrosis.[43,44] Liver disease may progress to biliary cirrhosis and portal hypertension in a minority of patients. The pathogenesis of liver disease in SBS is multifactorial; in infants, the risk is increased with prematurity, low birth weight, duration of parenteral nutrition, recurrent sepsis, and multiple laparotomies. In patients with no enteral feeding, decreased gut hormone secretion can cause biliary stasis and the development of biliary sludge and gallstones, which can further impair hepatic dysfunction. Deficiency of taurine, cysteine, and choline may also contribute to liver toxicity. Finally, conventional parenteral lipid solutions containing sunflower oil may also contribute to liver toxicity in these patients.

In SBS, liver disease usually presents with increasing jaundice, scleral icterus, hepato-splenomegaly, elevated serum transaminases, and eventually, portal hypertension. Monitoring of liver function tests is essential in the management of intestinal failure-associated liver disease . Doppler evaluation of hepatic and portal veins may be useful for assessment of portal hypertension. Liver biopsy is the gold standard to assess the extent of liver damage. Duro and colleagues[45] recently reported a noninvasive C13-methionine breath test to differentiate cirrhotic versus noncirrhotic patients.

MANAGEMENT OF SBS

Management of SBS requires a multidisciplinary approach that includes neonatologists, gastroenterologists, surgeons, nutritionists, pharmacists, nurses, and social workers. A cohesive, integrated multidisciplinary approach has been shown to increase rates of survival in children with SBS.[46] The aims of clinical management in SBS are to (1) provide sufficient nutrition to facilitate growth, (2) minimize fluid, nutritional, and electrolyte losses, and (3) maximize intestinal adaptation.

Parenteral Nutrition

Parenteral nutrition is used in infants with SBS to provide adequate caloric intake, macronutrients, and micronutrients to optimize growth and development. Parenteral nutrition should provide appropriate caloric intake to promote growth but avoid excessive weight gain without linear growth. Careful attention should be paid to protein intake to prevent catabolism, and some patients may need up to 3.5 g/kg/d.[47] Some authors have advocated restricting carbohydrates in the immediate perioperative period as many patients with SBS are unable to use these calories optimally during this period of stress.[38] To ensure optimal total caloric intake, fats comprise a critical part of parenteral nutrition. However, there is increasing concern that the cumulative amount of lipid in parenteral nutrition in patients with SBS is an independent risk factor for the development of cholestasis.[48]

Current lipid formulations are based on soybean lipids, olive oil lipids, or fish oil lipids. Patients on long-term parenteral nutrition are at increased risk of cholestasis, fatty liver, and hepatic fibrosis. Limiting soy lipid–based formulations to less than 0.5 g/kg/d has been shown to delay or even prevent cholestasis.[48] About 50% of the fatty acids present in soy-based formulations are the ω-6 polyunsaturated fatty acids, such as linoleic acid, which is a cause of concern because linoleic acid may have immunosuppressive and pro-inflammatory effects.[49] Soy lipid formulations have also been linked to impaired glucose homeostasis, where gluconeogenesis was increased but the normal reduction in glycogenolysis was inhibited.[50]

Fish oil–based formulations such as "Omegaven," which are rich in ω-3 fatty acids, have shown promise for reversing parenteral nutrition-associated cholestasis. This formulation is currently available in Europe and is an investigational drug in the United States. The efficacy and safety of fish oil lipid were evaluated in 19 infants who developed cholestasis while on soy lipid-based formula.[51] These patients were started on fish oil lipid–based formula and the soy lipid–based formula was discontinued. Compared with a historical cohort, infants on fish oil lipids showed reversal of cholestasis at 9.4 weeks, compared with 44.1 weeks in a historical cohort taking soy lipids and also had lower mortality. Administration of fish oil lipids was not associated with fatty acid deficiency, hypertriglyceridemia, infection, growth delay, or coagulopathy.[51] Similar findings were reported in other studies.[52–54]

Olive oil–based parenteral nutrition formulas have also been shown to be safe and well-tolerated in infants.[55] Compared to soy-lipid formulations, olive oil–based lipids contain lower levels of linoleic acid, thereby avoiding some of the adverse effects associated with ω-6 polyunsaturated fatty acids.[49] Furthermore, olive oil formulations do not seem to have the same effects on glucose metabolism that soy lipid formulations do.[50] Olive oil–based formulations can also decrease total cholesterol and low-density lipoproteins, with no significant differences in liver functions or adverse events.[55]

Patients with SBS need careful monitoring for electrolyte balance. Infants with ileostomy or poor colonic function can lose considerable amounts of sodium in stool. In the absence of adequate sodium replacement, compensatory hyperaldosteronism may ensue[56] and result in increased urinary potassium losses. Generally, parenteral sodium replacement is considered adequate if levels of urinary sodium are greater than 30 mEq/L.[38]

Trace element depletion is not unusual in patients with SBS on parenteral nutrition. Zinc is of particular importance in infants with extensive intestinal resection, as substantial amounts of zinc could be lost in ileostomy fluid (as high as 17 mg/L ileostomy fluid). Infants with SBS who are dependent on parenteral nutrition often require 300 to 500 μg/kg/d of zinc.[47]

Enteral Nutrition

There is little agreement in the literature regarding the timing of initiation or the rate of advancement of enteral feedings in SBS. Most clinicians prefer to start enteral feedings as soon as possible, hoping to promote intestinal adaptation, achieve full enteral feeds sooner, and prevent parenteral nutrition-associated adverse events.[2,38] In SBS, continuous administration of enteral nutrition is the preferred method because of a lower risk of osmotic diarrhea and an overall better tolerance than bolus feeds.[57]

The optimal formula of enteral feeds has not yet been established. Most clinicians prefer human milk or a semi-elemental or amino acid–based formula containing medium-chained and long-chained triglycerides.[38,58] In experimental models, formulations containing complex proteins, disaccharides, and long-chain triglycerides increased intestinal adaptation, but concerns remain about increased gut permeability to complex proteins and the risk of sensitization. Human breast milk is associated with a shorter duration of parenteral nutrition when compared with cow's milk or protein hydrolysates.[26] The difference between hydrolyzed protein and nonhydrolyzed protein has been evaluated in infants receiving some enteral and parenteral nutrition, and no difference was noted in energy intake, intestinal permeability, or nitrogen balance.[59]

The rate of advancement of enteral feedings should be individualized with careful monitoring of stool/stoma output, vomiting, and abdominal distention. Generally, stool/stoma output should be limited to 40 to 50 mL/kg/d, although higher outputs may be permissible if hydration, acid-base status, and electrolyte balance can be maintained.[47] The authors typically increase enteral feedings to volumes whereby the stool output is at maximally tolerated levels, and then as the bowel adapts, increase the volume and/or concentration of feeds.[58]

PHARMACOLOGIC INTERVENTIONS IN SBS
Acid Suppressing Agents

Patients with SBS frequently develop hypergastrinemia, which leads to increased gastric acid secretion. H_2-receptor blockers and proton pump inhibitors are often used to suppress gastric acid secretion, especially for the first 6 months after surgery.

Prokinetic Agents

Intestinal dysmotility is an important cause of morbidity in patients with SBS.[60] Symptoms of intestinal dysmotility include abdominal distention, vomiting, feeding intolerance, and inability to make progress on enteral feeds. Bacterial overgrowth, lactic acidosis, bacterial translocation, and systemic infection are complications of intestinal dysmotility and distension. Various pharmacologic agents have been used to treat intestinal dysmotility.

Erythromycin
Erythromycin increases gut motility by activating motilin receptors. In physiologic studies, prokinetic effects of erythromycin are observed at doses as low as 10 to 20 mg/kg/d. However, in a systematic review examining 10 randomized controlled studies, both high-dose and low-dose erythromycin failed to show improvement in feeding intolerance in preterm infants.[61] In a recent review,[62] erythromycin use was associated with shorter time to full feeds, decreased duration of parenteral nutrition, and decreased incidence of cholestasis.

Metoclopramide
Metoclopramide, a dopamine receptor antagonist with moderate serotonergic activity, can improve lower esophageal sphincter tone, improve gastric emptying, and facilitate antropyloroduodenal contractions. Adverse effects of metoclopramide include extrapyramidal reactions in up to 30% patients. In 2009, the Food and Drug Administration added labeling changes including limiting metoclopramide use to less than 12 weeks.

Data on use of metoclopramide in SBS patients are limited.[60] When used, metoclopramide is given enterally at a dose of 0.1 mg/kg 3 to 4 times a day for 2 to 3 weeks.

Anti-diarrheal agents
Anti-diarrheal agents are used to reduce gut motility in selected patients with high ostomies:

Opioid agents
Opioid agents decrease peristalsis, increase absorption of fluid and electrolytes, increase tone in the large intestine, and increase anal sphincter tone. In pediatric SBS, loperamide, diphenoxylate/atropine, and opium alkaloid codeine have been tried, although no data are available to compare these agents in children. Loperamide may be superior to codeine in reducing electrolyte losses and is the preferred agent to treat diarrhea in these patients.[60]

Absorbent agents
Absorbent agents, such as pectin and guar gum agents, act by absorbing fluids and compounds and binding potential intestinal toxins from the gut. These agents can reduce the intestinal transit time and reduce diarrhea.[63] Caution should be used in patients with significant dysmotility as it may lead to bacterial overgrowth and lactic acidosis.[60]

Ursodeoxycholic acid (UDCA)
UDCA is a hydrophilic derivative of chenodeoxycholic acid, which acts by displacing endogenous, more hydrophobic, toxic bile acids. UDCA can arrest rising alkaline phosphatase and also lower levels of serum bilirubin in patients with SBS and cholestasis.[64] UDCA is usually initiated orally at a dose of 20 mg/kg/d divided in 2 doses and is given for a period of 4 to 6 weeks.

Cholestyramine
In patients with SBS, particularly those with loss of ileum, there is a disruption of enterohepatic circulation of bile acids.[65] Unabsorbed bile acids reach the colon and cause irritation, leading to secretory diarrhea. Cholestyramine is beneficial in the treatment of bile acid–induced secretory diarrhea.[60]

Pharmacologic Approaches to Enhance Intestinal Adaptation

Various pharmacologic agents have been studied to accelerate intestinal adaptation in animal models and humans. Epidermal growth factor, growth hormone, GLP2, keratinocyte growth factor, and insulin-like growth factor 1 have been studied in animal models. Growth hormone and GLP2 have been studied in humans.[38] Growth hormone in combination with glucagon has shown some improvement in intestinal function in adults but has not been evaluated in pediatric SBS. A GLP-2 analogue (teduglutide) has been shown to reduce the need for parenteral nutrition by more than 20% in double-blind randomized human trials.[66]

SURGICAL MANAGEMENT OF SBS

Surgical interventions in SBS include bowel conservation at the time of initial presentation, bowel lengthening operations, and intestinal transplantation.

Bowel Conservation

The goal of the initial surgical procedure is to limit bowel loss and excise only the obviously compromised bowel. Any bowel of marginal viability is kept in situ.

A "second-look" procedure in 24 hours can be used to assess the viability of the remaining bowel.[2] During this period, a temporary "silo" can be used to prevent abdominal compartment syndrome, and closure can be performed once intestinal edema has resolved.

Longitudinal Intestinal Lengthening and Tailoring (LILT) Procedure

The LILT procedure was first described by Bianchi in 1980.[67] This procedure involves splitting the intestine into 2 longitudinal halves, and then anastomosing the halves in series with the rest of the intestine. This procedure doubles the length of the bowel and, at the same time, improves transit time and peristalsis by decreasing the diameter of the dilated bowel. All mucosae are preserved. However, there is no increase in the absorptive surface area. A modification of LILT was described in 1998,[68] whereby the intestine was divided in the middle of the dilated segment and staples were placed obliquely, then longitudinally, and then obliquely again to the opposite edge of the intestine. This procedure resulted in 2 intestinal segments that remained connected to the proximal and distal ends of the intestine. The free ends were then anastomosed. Only 1 anastomosis was needed, as opposed to 3 anastomoses in the original LILT procedure.[68]

The LILT procedure can be technically challenging; complications include fistula formation, anastomotic stenosis, and anastomotic leakage.[69,70] A high incidence of sepsis, progressive intestinal failure, and surgical complications has also been reported.[71] In a review of 20 patients,[72] 6-year rates of survival were 45%. Survivors had residual bowel length greater than 40 cm and no liver disease, whereas the non-survivors had shorter bowel lengths and significant cholestasis. The Bianchi procedure is not recommended in neonates, those with liver disease, or those with intestine length less than 50 cm.[71]

Serial Transverse Enteroplasty (STEP)

The STEP procedure was first described in 2003.[73] This procedure involves the application of surgical staples in a transmesenteric transverse fashion, which creates a longer and narrower intestinal lumen.[74] The STEP procedure has several advantages over the Bianchi procedure in being less technically challenging, resulting in a uniform lumen and in the ability to be repeated if redilatation of the bowel occurs.[75,76]

Outcomes from the STEP procedure have been encouraging. In a series of 38 patients,[74] the average increase in intestinal length was 69% and enteral caloric intake was noted to increase from 31% to 67% in a median 1-year period. Complications included staple line leak and intraoperative aspiration, bowel obstruction, hypertension, hematoma, abscess, and pleural effusions. Three patients died and another 3 received transplantation beyond 30 days postoperatively.[74] Similar results have been reported elsewhere.[77,78] In a group of 14 children who underwent the STEP procedure in Toronto, Canada, the total increase in intestinal length was 49%.[78] Parenteral nutrition calories decreased from 71% to 36% within 1 month and to 12% after 1 year. Compared with patients who underwent LILT, the STEP procedure allowed faster weaning off of parenteral nutrition and lower need for later transplants. No difference was found in early complications, growth rates, or survival rates.[70]

Intestinal Transplantation

Transplantation is a treatment of last resort, indicated mainly in patients with irreversible hepatic and intestinal failure.[79–81] With improved parenteral nutrition and consequent prevention of liver disease, the need for transplants has decreased.[2] Types of transplantation include isolated intestine, isolated liver, combined liver and intestine, and multivisceral. Current indications for intestinal transplantation, combined intestine/liver transplantation, or multivisceral transplantation for patients with irreversible intestinal failure are as follows: (1) impending liver failure as manifested by jaundice, elevated liver injury tests, clinical findings (splenomegaly, varices, coagulopathy), history of stomal bleeding, or hepatic cirrhosis on biopsy; (2) loss of major venous access defined as more than 2 thromboses in the great vessels (subclavian, jugular, and femoral veins); (3) frequent central line–related sepsis consisting of more than 2 episodes of systemic sepsis per year, or 1 episode of line-related fungemia; (4) recurrent episodes of severe dehydration despite intravenous fluid management.[82] Complications of transplantation include acute rejection, infection, graft-versus-host disease, and posttransplant lymphoproliferative disease. Factors contributing to poor outcomes include multiple pretransplant surgeries, end-stage liver disease, inferior vena cava thrombosis, and hospitalization versus home care.[83] One-year patient and intestine graft survival is 89% and 79% for intestine-only recipients and 72% and 69% for liver-intestine recipients, respectively. By 10 years, patient and intestine graft survival decreases to 46% and 29% for intestine-only recipients, and 42% and 39% for liver-intestine recipients, respectively.[79] More recently, living donor intestinal transplantation and combined living donor intestine/liver transplant have been performed successfully in pediatric patients with intestinal and liver failure and have a major advantage of virtually eliminating waiting time.[80,84]

SUMMARY

SBS is the most common cause of intestinal failure in infants. Advancements in parenteral nutrition, strategies to prevent infections, surgical technique, and intestinal transplantation have greatly increased survival in patients with SBS. With a cohesive and integrated management plan and a multidisciplinary approach, most neonates with SBS can be transitioned to enteral feeding and to achieve normal growth and development.

REFERENCES

1. Goulet O, Ruemmele F. Causes and management of intestinal failure in children. Gastroenterology 2006;130:S16–28.
2. Gutierrez IM, Kang KH, Jaksic T. Neonatal short bowel syndrome. Semin Fetal Neonatal Med 2011;16:157–63.
3. Wales PW, Christison-Lagay ER. Short bowel syndrome: epidemiology and etiology. Semin Pediatr Surg 2010;19:3–9.
4. Cole CR, Hansen NI, Higgins RD, et al. Very low birth weight preterm infants with surgical short bowel syndrome: incidence, morbidity and mortality, and growth outcomes at 18 to 22 months. Pediatrics 2008;122:e573–82.
5. Wales PW, de Silva N, Kim J, et al. Neonatal short bowel syndrome: population-based estimates of incidence and mortality rates. J Pediatr Surg 2004;39:690–5.
6. Salvia G, Guarino A, Terrin G, et al. Neonatal onset intestinal failure: an Italian Multicenter Study. J Pediatr 2008;153:674–6, 676.e1–2.
7. Mazariegos GV, Squires RH, Sindhi RK. Current perspectives on pediatric intestinal transplantation. Curr Gastroenterol Rep 2009;11:226–33.
8. Duro D, Kalish LA, Johnston P, et al. Risk factors for intestinal failure in infants with necrotizing enterocolitis: a Glaser Pediatric Research Network study. J Pediatr 2010;157:203–208.e201.

9. Squires RH, Duggan C, Teitelbaum DH, et al. Natural history of pediatric intestinal failure: initial report from the pediatric intestinal failure consortium. J Pediatr 2012; 161(4):723–728.e2.

10. Chabra S, Gleason CA, Seidel K, et al. Rising prevalence of gastroschisis in Washington State. J Toxicol Environ Health A 2011;74:336–45.

11. Vu LT, Nobuhara KK, Laurent C, et al. Increasing prevalence of gastroschisis: population-based study in California. J Pediatr 2008;152:807–11.

12. Trobs RB, Tannapfel A. Apple peel small bowel. Imaging case book. J Perinatol 2009;29:832–3.

13. Festen S, Brevoord JC, Goldhoorn GA, et al. Excellent long-term outcome for survivors of apple peel atresia. J Pediatr Surg 2002;37:61–5.

14. Sapin E, Carricaburu E, De Boissieu D, et al. Conservative intestinal surgery to avoid short-bowel syndrome in multiple intestinal atresias and necrotizing entero-colitis: 6 cases treated by multiple anastomoses and Santulli-type enterostomy. Eur J Pediatr Surg 1999;9:24–8.

15. Sapin E, Joyeux L. Multiple intestinal anastomoses to avoid short bowel syndrome and stimulate bowel maturity in type IV multiple intestinal atresia and necrotizing enterocolitis. J Pediatr Surg 2012;47:628.

16. Laughlin DM, Friedmacher F, Puri P. Total colonic aganglionosis: a systematic review and meta-analysis of long-term clinical outcome. Pediatr Surg Int 2012;28:773–9.

17. Elhalaby EA, Teitelbaum DH, Coran AG, et al. Enterocolitis associated with Hirschsprung's disease: a clinical histopathological correlative study. J Pediatr Surg 1995;30:1023–6 [discussion: 1026–7].

18. Finkel Y, Goulet O. Short bowel syndrome. In: Kleinman RE, Sanderson IR, Goulet O, et al, editors. Walker's pediatric gastrointestinal disease. Hamilton (Ontario): BC Decker, Inc; 2008. p. 601–12.

19. Serrano MS, Schmidt-Sommerfeld E. Nutrition support of infants with short bowel syndrome. Nutrition 2002;18:966–70.

20. Sukhotnik I, Siplovich L, Shiloni E, et al. Intestinal adaptation in short-bowel syndrome in infants and children: a collective review. Pediatr Surg Int 2002;18:258–63.

21. Sidhu GS, Narasimharao KL, Rani VU, et al. Morphological and functional changes in the gut after massive small bowel resection and colon interposition in rhesus monkeys. Digestion 1984;29:47–54.

22. Spencer AU, Neaga A, West B, et al. Pediatric short bowel syndrome: redefining predictors of success. Ann Surg 2005;242:403–9 [discussion: 409–12].

23. Struijs MC, Diamond IR, de Silva N, et al. Establishing norms for intestinal length in children. J Pediatr Surg 2009;44:933–8.

24. Touloukian RJ, Smith GJ. Normal intestinal length in preterm infants. J Pediatr Surg 1983;18:720–3.

25. Koffeman GI, van Gemert WG, George EK, et al. Classification, epidemiology and aetiology. Best Pract Res Clin Gastroenterol 2003;17:879–93.

26. Andorsky DJ, Lund DP, Lillehei CW, et al. Nutritional and other postoperative management of neonates with short bowel syndrome correlates with clinical outcomes. J Pediatr 2001;139:27–33.

27. Wilmore DW. Factors correlating with a successful outcome following extensive intestinal resection in newborn infants. J Pediatr 1972;80:88–95.

28. Buchman AL, Scolapio J, Fryer J. AGA technical review on short bowel syndrome and intestinal transplantation. Gastroenterology 2003;124:1111–34.

29. Nightingale JM, Kamm MA, van der Sijp JR, et al. Gastrointestinal hormones in short bowel syndrome. Peptide YY may be the 'colonic brake' to gastric emptying. Gut 1996;39:267–72.

30. Crenn P, Coudray-Lucas C, Cynober L, et al. Post-absorptive plasma citrulline concentration: a marker of intestinal failure in humans. Transplant Proc 1998;30:2528.
31. Diamanti A, Panetta F, Gandullia P, et al. Plasma citrulline as marker of bowel adaptation in children with short bowel syndrome. Langenbecks Arch Surg 2011;396:1041–6.
32. Rhoads JM, Plunkett E, Galanko J, et al. Serum citrulline levels correlate with enteral tolerance and bowel length in infants with short bowel syndrome. J Pediatr 2005;146:542–7.
33. Fitzgibbons S, Ching YA, Valim C, et al. Relationship between serum citrulline levels and progression to parenteral nutrition independence in children with short bowel syndrome. J Pediatr Surg 2009;44:928–32.
34. Casaccia G, Trucchi A, Spirydakis I, et al. Congenital intestinal anomalies, neonatal short bowel syndrome, and prenatal/neonatal counseling. J Pediatr Surg 2006;41:804–7.
35. Wales PW, de Silva N, Kim JH, et al. Neonatal short bowel syndrome: a cohort study. J Pediatr Surg 2005;40:755–62.
36. Hyman PE, Everett SL, Harada T. Gastric acid hypersecretion in short bowel syndrome in infants: association with extent of resection and enteral feeding. J Pediatr Gastroenterol Nutr 1986;5:191–7.
37. Williams NS, Evans P, King RF. Gastric acid secretion and gastrin production in the short bowel syndrome. Gut 1985;26:914–9.
38. Kocoshis SA. Medical management of pediatric intestinal failure. Semin Pediatr Surg 2010;19:20–6.
39. Bongaerts G, Tolboom J, Naber T, et al. D-lactic acidemia and aciduria in pediatric and adult patients with short bowel syndrome. Clin Chem 1995;41:107–10.
40. Schimpl G, Feierl G, Linni K, et al. Bacterial translocation in short-bowel syndrome in rats. Eur J Pediatr Surg 1999;9:224–7.
41. Jones BA, Hull MA, Richardson DS, et al. Efficacy of ethanol locks in reducing central venous catheter infections in pediatric patients with intestinal failure. J Pediatr Surg 2010;45:1287–93.
42. Mouw E, Chessman K, Lesher A, et al. Use of an ethanol lock to prevent catheter-related infections in children with short bowel syndrome. J Pediatr Surg 2008;43:1025–9.
43. Kelly DA. Intestinal failure-associated liver disease: what do we know today? Gastroenterology 2006;130:S70–7.
44. Kelly DA. Preventing parenteral nutrition liver disease. Early Hum Dev 2010;86:683–7.
45. Duro D, Fitzgibbons S, Valim C, et al. [13C]Methionine breath test to assess intestinal failure-associated liver disease. Pediatr Res 2010;68:349–54.
46. Modi BP, Langer M, Ching YA, et al. Improved survival in a multidisciplinary short bowel syndrome program. J Pediatr Surg 2008;43:20–4.
47. Wessel JJ, Kocoshis SA. Nutritional management of infants with short bowel syndrome. Semin Perinatol 2007;31:104–11.
48. Shin JI, Namgung R, Park MS, et al. Could lipid infusion be a risk for parenteral nutrition-associated cholestasis in low birth weight neonates? Eur J Pediatr 2008;167:197–202.
49. Sala-Vila A, Barbosa VM, Calder PC. Olive oil in parenteral nutrition. Curr Opin Clin Nutr Metab Care 2007;10:165–74.
50. van Kempen AA, van der Crabben SN, Ackermans MT, et al. Stimulation of gluconeogenesis by intravenous lipids in preterm infants: response depends on fatty acid profile. Am J Physiol Endocrinol Metab 2006;290:E723–30.

51. Gura KM, Lee S, Valim C, et al. Safety and efficacy of a fish-oil-based fat emulsion in the treatment of parenteral nutrition-associated liver disease. Pediatrics 2008; 121:e678–86.
52. Chung PH, Wong KK, Wong RM, et al. Clinical experience in managing pediatric patients with ultra-short bowel syndrome using omega-3 fatty acid. Eur J Pediatr Surg 2010;20:139–42.
53. Diamond IR, Sterescu A, Pencharz PB, et al. Changing the paradigm: omegaven for the treatment of liver failure in pediatric short bowel syndrome. J Pediatr Gastroenterol Nutr 2009;48:209–15.
54. Puder M, Valim C, Meisel JA, et al. Parenteral fish oil improves outcomes in patients with parenteral nutrition-associated liver injury. Ann Surg 2009;250: 395–402.
55. Goulet O, de Potter S, Antebi H, et al. Long-term efficacy and safety of a new olive oil-based intravenous fat emulsion in pediatric patients: a double-blind randomized study. Am J Clin Nutr 1999;70:338–45.
56. Schwarz KB, Ternberg JL, Bell MJ, et al. Sodium needs of infants and children with ileostomy. J Pediatr 1983;102:509–13.
57. Vanderhoof JA, Matya SM. Enteral and parenteral nutrition in patients with short-bowel syndrome. Eur J Pediatr Surg 1999;9:214–9.
58. Rudolph JA, Squires R. Current concepts in the medical management of pediatric intestinal failure. Curr Opin Organ Transplant 2010;15:324–9.
59. Ksiazyk J, Piena M, Kierkus J, et al. Hydrolyzed versus nonhydrolyzed protein diet in short bowel syndrome in children. J Pediatr Gastroenterol Nutr 2002;35:615–8.
60. Dicken BJ, Sergi C, Rescorla FJ, et al. Medical management of motility disorders in patients with intestinal failure: a focus on necrotizing enterocolitis, gastroschisis, and intestinal atresia. J Pediatr Surg 2011;46:1618–30.
61. Ng E, Shah VS. Erythromycin for the prevention and treatment of feeding intolerance in preterm infants. Cochrane Database Syst Rev 2008;(3):CD001815.
62. Ng PC. Use of oral erythromycin for the treatment of gastrointestinal dysmotility in preterm infants. Neonatology 2009;95:97–104.
63. Drenckpohl D, Hocker J, Shareef M, et al. Adding dietary green beans resolves the diarrhea associated with bowel surgery in neonates: a case study. Nutr Clin Pract 2005;20:674–7.
64. De Marco G, Sordino D, Bruzzese E, et al. Early treatment with ursodeoxycholic acid for cholestasis in children on parenteral nutrition because of primary intestinal failure. Aliment Pharmacol Ther 2006;24:387–94.
65. Sinha L, Liston R, Testa HJ, et al. Idiopathic bile acid malabsorption: qualitative and quantitative clinical features and response to cholestyramine. Aliment Pharmacol Ther 1998;12:839–44.
66. Jeppesen PB, Gilroy R, Pertkiewicz M, et al. Randomised placebo-controlled trial of teduglutide in reducing parenteral nutrition and/or intravenous fluid requirements in patients with short bowel syndrome. Gut 2011;60:902–14.
67. Bianchi A. Intestinal loop lengthening–a technique for increasing small intestinal length. J Pediatr Surg 1980;15:145–51.
68. Chahine AA, Ricketts RR. A modification of the Bianchi intestinal lengthening procedure with a single anastomosis. J Pediatr Surg 1998;33:1292–3.
69. Huskisson LJ, Brereton RJ, Kiely EM, et al. Problems with intestinal lengthening. J Pediatr Surg 1993;28:720–2.
70. Sudan D, Thompson J, Botha J, et al. Comparison of intestinal lengthening procedures for patients with short bowel syndrome. Ann Surg 2007;246:593–601 [discussion: 601–4].

71. Bueno J, Guiterrez J, Mazariegos GV, et al. Analysis of patients with longitudinal intestinal lengthening procedure referred for intestinal transplantation. J Pediatr Surg 2001;36:178–83.

72. Bianchi A. Longitudinal intestinal lengthening and tailoring: results in 20 children. J R Soc Med 1997;90:429–32.

73. Kim HB, Fauza D, Garza J, et al. Serial transverse enteroplasty (STEP): a novel bowel lengthening procedure. J Pediatr Surg 2003;38:425–9.

74. Modi BP, Javid PJ, Jaksic T, et al. First report of the international serial transverse enteroplasty data registry: indications, efficacy, and complications. J Am Coll Surg 2007;204:365–71.

75. Ehrlich PF, Mychaliska GB, Teitelbaum DH. The 2 STEP: an approach to repeating a serial transverse enteroplasty. J Pediatr Surg 2007;42:819–22.

76. Morikawa N, Kuroda T, Kitano Y. Repeat STEP procedure to establish enteral nutrition in an infant with short bowel syndrome. Pediatr Surg Int 2009;25: 1007–11.

77. Javid PJ, Kim HB, Duggan CP, et al. Serial transverse enteroplasty is associated with successful short-term outcomes in infants with short bowel syndrome. J Pediatr Surg 2005;40:1019–23 [discussion: 1023–4].

78. Wales PW, de Silva N, Langer JC, et al. Intermediate outcomes after serial transverse enteroplasty in children with short bowel syndrome. J Pediatr Surg 2007;42: 1804–10.

79. Mazariegos GV, Steffick DE, Horslen S, et al. Intestine transplantation in the United States, 1999-2008. Am J Transplant 2010;10:1020–34.

80. Tzvetanov IG, Oberholzer J, Benedetti E. Current status of living donor small bowel transplantation. Curr Opin Organ Transplant 2010;15:346–8.

81. Ueno T, Wada M, Hoshino K, et al. Current status of intestinal transplantation in Japan. Transplant Proc 2011;43:2405–7.

82. Mazariegos GV. Intestinal transplantation: current outcomes and opportunities. Curr Opin Organ Transplant 2009;14:515–21.

83. Sauvat F, Dupic L, Caldari D, et al. Factors influencing outcome after intestinal transplantation in children. Transplant Proc 2006;38:1689–91.

84. Berg CL, Steffick DE, Edwards EB, et al. Liver and intestine transplantation in the United States 1998-2007. Am J Transplant 2009;9:907–31.

Necrotizing Enterocolitis in Term Infants

Robert D. Christensen, MD[a],*, Diane K. Lambert, RN[a],
Vickie L. Baer, RN[a], Phillip V. Gordon, MD[b]

KEYWORDS

- Necrotizing enterocolitis • Term-NEC • Risk factors • Human milk
- Narcotic withdrawal

KEY POINTS

- Necrotizing enterocolitis in term neonates is not a primary diagnosis; rather, it occurs among a subset of neonates admitted to a neonatal intensive care unit for some other illness or condition.
- Features predisposing term neonates to necrotizing enterocolitis include reduced mesenteric perfusion, as occurs with polycythemia or sepsis.
- In recent years, term necrotizing enterocolitis has been recognized among neonates undergoing abstinence from maternal opioid narcotics.
- Term necrotizing enterocolitis generally occurs among those with predisposing gastrointestinal pathology who are fed cow's milk–based formulas in volumes much greater than similar-aged breast feeding neonates receive.

INTRODUCTION

Necrotizing enterocolitis (NEC) occurs primarily among prematurely delivered infants, with an incidence inversely proportional to gestational age at birth.[1] NEC is uncommon among full-term infants, although this has been well described in multiple reports.[2–16] Most publications of term NEC are individual case reports or small case series, owing to the rarity of this condition at individual institutions.

In 2007 the authors reported on 30 term neonates with NEC from the Intermountain Healthcare hospitals.[17,18] This was the largest cases series of NEC in term infants of which we were aware. These 30 were born in the 5½-year period from January 1, 2001 through June 30, 2006. In this article, the authors review these 30 and summarize the

Disclosures: None of the authors has a conflict of interest with regard to this study or manuscript.
[a] The Women and Newborns Program, Intermountain Healthcare, Salt Lake City, Ogden, UT 84111, USA; [b] The Division of Neonatology, Department of Pediatrics, Tulane University School of Medicine, New Orleans, LA 70112, USA
* Corresponding author. NICU, McKay-Dee Hospital Center, 4th Floor, 4401 Harrison Boulevard, Ogden, UT 84403.
E-mail address: Robert.christensen@imail.org

Clin Perinatol 40 (2013) 69–78
http://dx.doi.org/10.1016/j.clp.2012.12.007
0095-5108/13/$ – see front matter © 2013 Elsevier Inc. All rights reserved.

characteristics of another 23 born in the period from July 1, 2006 through December 31, 2011. Whereas most infants in whom NEC developed during the first epoch were admitted to the neonatal intensive care unit (NICU) for another reason such as congenital heart disease, polycythemia, or sepsis, we have encountered several infants in whom NEC developed while undergoing withdrawal from maternal opioid narcotics.

FINDINGS IN THE FIRST EPOCH (2001–2006)

During the first period studied, the Intermountain Healthcare NICUs admitted 11,523 neonates, and, of these, 5877 (51%) were greater than 36 weeks' gestation at birth. Thirty of these went on to have NEC Bell's stage $\geq$II.[19–21] NEC was defined by the presence of one or more of the following 3 clinical signs: (1) bilious gastric aspirate or emesis, (2) abdominal distension, (3) occult or gross blood in stool (no fissure), and one or more of the following 3 radiographic findings; (1) pneumatosis intestinalis, (2) hepatobiliary gas, (3) pneumoperitoneum. If a patient had focal gastrointestinal perforation, based on visual inspection of the bowel at the time of surgery or postmortem examination, the condition was not listed as NEC but as a focal gastrointestinal perforation. In our analysis of these 30,[17] we judged that 3 findings were of potential importance in identifying the pathogenic mechanism: (1) NEC occurred exclusively among neonates already admitted to the NICU for some other reason. Thus, NEC was invariably a complication of treatment as opposed to a presenting problem. (2) Certain diagnoses, at the time of admission to the NICU, were statistically more common among those who went on to have NEC. Foremost among these were congenital heart disease (particularly ductal-dependent varieties), polycythemia, and early-onset sepsis. The authors speculated that these disorders predisposed to NEC based on reduced mesenteric perfusion. (3) This variety of NEC was much more common if the neonate was fed cow's milk–based formulas, particularly if large-volume feedings were administered (compared with the amounts usually ingested by breast-feeding neonates in the first days after birth).[22]

The authors proposed that these 3 features could be united into a common pathogenesis; namely, neonates admitted to an NICU with conditions involving reduced mesenteric perfusion and fed large volumes of cow's milk formulas in the first days. Clearly, NEC developed in only a minority of neonates with these features; thus, these features were not sufficient to cause the disease. However, they were so common among the 30 in whom term NEC developed as to suggest that they were necessary, although not sufficient, for causation. On this basis, we speculated that when term neonates are admitted to the NICU with conditions likely resulting in reduced mesenteric perfusion, care should be taken not to overfeed them using cow's milk–based formulas.[17,18]

FINDINGS IN THE SECOND EPOCH (2006–2011)

During the second period studied, the Intermountain Healthcare NICUs admitted 11,504 neonates, and, of these, 5719 (50%) were greater than 36 weeks of gestation at delivery. Twenty-two of these went on to have NEC Bell's stage $\geq$II. As in the first epoch, NEC occurred exclusively among those who had been admitted to an NICU for some other reason. Thus, in these patients too, NEC was a complication of NICU care.

Table 1 shows the diagnoses, at the time of NICU admission, for these 52 neonates. In both epochs, the most common admitting diagnoses were respiratory distress, suspected congenital heart disease, and infection/sepsis/shock. In the second epoch, 9 of the 22 were undergoing management for withdrawal from opioid narcotics during pregnancy. No similar cases were observed during the first epoch.

Table 1
Diagnoses on admission to the NICU of neonates who went on to have NEC in 2 consecutive 5½-year periods

	Period 1		Period 2		
Admission Diagnosis	Admitted to the NICU (n = 5877)	NEC Developed Subsequently (n = 30)	Admitted to the NICU (n = 5719)	NEC Developed Subsequently (n = 22)	P Value Period 1 vs 2
Respiratory distress	1929	8 (0.4%)	1999	2 (0.1%)	.049
Suspected infection	1102	0	684	3 (0.4%)	.028
Suspected or proven congenital heart disease	534	8 (1.5%)	364	4 (1.1%)	NS
Hypoglycemia	446	0	626	2 (0.3%)	NS
Gastroschisis-omphalo-TEF-imperforate anus	185	0	100	1 (1%)	NS
Aspiration	158	0	177	0	NS
Jaundice	126	0	114	0	NS
Transient tachypnea	123	0	87	0	NS
Seizures	63	0	27	0	NS
Birth depression	43	4 (9%)	68	0	.014
Pulmonary hypertension	38	0	18	0	NS
Pneumothorax	29	0	26	0	NS
Shock/sepsis	16	8 (50%)	36	1 (3%)	**.002**
Polycythemia	15	2 (13%)	4	0	NS
Withdrawal from maternal opioid narcotics	63	0	102	9 (9%)	.015
Other	1070	0	1287	0	NS

Period 1 is January 2001–June 2006, and period 2 is July 2006–December 2011. (Bonferroni adjustment: Lower the P value of .05 to .0036).

Abbreviations: NS, not significant; TEC, tracheoesophageal fistula; bolded P-values indicate the finding remained significant after Bonferroni's correction.

Table 2 shows the final diagnoses for these 52 compared with a cohort of term neonates admitted to the same NICUs who did not have NEC. In the first epoch, congenital heart disease and polycythemia conveyed a risk for NEC. These associations were not evident in the second period (after the Bonferroni correction). In both epochs, no associations were identified based on race, Apgar score, gender, or maternal age.

Table 3 shows elements of the hospital course among the term neonates with NEC. In the second epoch, cases presented somewhat earlier than in the first, and survival was better.

COMPARISON OF THE NEONATES WITH NEC IN THE 2 EPOCHS

The incidence of NEC was 5.1 and 3.8 cases per 1000 term neonates admitted to the NICU during the first and second epochs, respectively. However, in the second epoch, 9 cases of a new variety of NEC were observed, not previously identified in our

Table 2
Discharge diagnoses and features of neonates that developed NEC versus others that did not develop NEC but were of the same gestational age range and cared for in the same NICUs during the same period of time

Final Diagnoses and Features	Period 1			Period 2		
	Developed NEC (n = 30)	Did not Develop NEC (n = 5847)	P Value	Developed NEC (n = 22)	Did not Develop NEC (n = 5697)	P Value
Congenital heart disease	27% (8)	5% (270)	**.000**	18% (4)	(6%) 336	**.015**
Polycythemia	7% (2)	0.2% (13)	**.002**	0% (0)	0.7% (4)	.901
Early-onset bacterial sepsis	13% (4)	2% (131)	**.004**	9% (2)	2% (111)	**.016**
Birth weight (g)	2849 ± 581	3180 ± 594	**.010**	3287 ± 831	3155 ± 603	.300
Endotracheal intubation	60% (18)	41% (2395)	.028	36% (8)	34% (1943)	.824
PDA	23% (7)	15% (867)	.081	18% (4)	15% (849)	.666
On vasopressors	20% (6)	12% (724)	.090	14% (3)	14% (813)	.932
Maternal antenatal corticosteroids	7% (2)	2% (137)	.125	14% (3)	5% (283)	.062
Aspiration	7% (2)	3% (151)	.141	5% (1)	3% (176)	.694
Maternal cigarette smoking	3% (1)	10% (564)	.153	23% (5)	12% (515)	.026
Non-White race	20% (6)	17% (997)	.165	23% (5)	12% (687)	.126
Gestational age at birth (wk)	37.6 ± 1.4	38.2 ± 1.4	NS	38.5 ± 1.4	38.0 ± 1.4	.388
Apgar (1 min)	6.9 ± 2.0	6.7 ± 2.2	NS	6.9 ± 2.3	6.8 ± 3.9	.916
Apgar (5 min)	8.2 ± 1.5	8.1 ± 1.5	NS	8.4 ± 1.0	8.2 ± 2.8	.805
Gender (percent male)	53% (16)	59% (3438)	NS	64% (14)	60% (3437)	.752
Maternal Age (y)	26.9 ± 6.0	26.9 ± 5.6	NS	27.4 ± 5.5	27.7 ± 5.5	.798

Neonates in 2 consecutive 5½-year periods are shown; period 1 is January 2001–June 2006, period 2 is July 2006–December 2011. (Bonferroni adjustment: Lower the P value of .05 to .003).

Abbreviation: NS, not significant; bolded P-values indicate the finding remained significant after Bonferroni's correction.

Table 3
Hospital course of NEC among 52 term neonates

Hospital Course	Period 1 Mean ± SD; or (Median; Range); or [%]	Period 2 Mean ± SD; or (Median; Range); or [%]	P Value Period 1 vs 2
Age (d) when NEC was diagnosed	15 ± 12 (12; 1–46)	8 ± 7 (6; 2–24)	.011
Location of patient when NEC developed	Home = 2[a]; WBN = 0; NICU = 28	Home = 0; WBN = 0; NICU = 22	.502
Transferred to children's hospital for surgical management	8 [27]	3 [14]	.319
Surgery for NEC	7 [23]	3 [14]	.488
Bowel perforation and resection	5 [17]	3 [14]	1.000
Total bowel necrosis	2 [7]	0 [0]	.502
Survival (%)	26/30 [87]	21/22 [95]	.011
Length of hospital stay (d) among survivors	(37; 7–145)	(31; 16–91)	.736

Neonates in 2 consecutive 5½-year periods are shown; period 1 was January 2001–June 2006, and period 2 was July 2006–December 2011.
Abbreviation: WBN, well baby nursery.
[a] Two patients developed NEC at home, but both had been discharged from an NICU one day (first case) or 2 days (second case) before the NEC was recognized. Both cases had bloody stools and abdominal distention occurring at home, prompting hospital readmission.

databases; namely, NEC among neonates undergoing managed withdrawal from maternal opioid narcotics. With these 9 cases excluded from the incidence figures, the incidence during the second epoch was 2.3 per 1000, which was significantly lower than that in the first epoch (P = .009). There was a significant reduction in NEC among those with an admitting diagnosis of shock and sepsis. There were other trends that did not reach statistical significance, including reductions in NEC associated with respiratory distress and birth asphyxia. We found a significant increase in term NEC associated with narcotic withdrawal.

In the first period, NEC was recognized, on average, on day-of-life 15. In the second period, it was recognized, on average, on day-of-life 8 (*see* **Table 3**). This difference was influenced by the more rapid development of NEC in the subgroup with narcotic withdrawal. Those 9 had NEC diagnosed on an average of day 8.7.

NEC AMONG NEONATES UNDERGOING WITHDRAWAL FROM MATERNAL OPIOID NARCOTICS

Features of the 9 in whom NEC developed while being treated for withdrawal from maternal opioids are provided in **Table 4**. These 9 were cared for in 5 different hospitals in various parts of the state. Five were small for gestational age. During pregnancy, 4 of the 9 mothers were receiving Suboxone and 5 were receiving methadone. All but one was fed a standard cow's milk–based formula. Although these were all term infants, 5 were primarily receiving gavage feedings because of agitation and poor nippling as part of the withdrawal symptoms.

Patrick and colleagues[23] recently reported a nationwide database search of neonatal abstinence syndrome showing a marked increase in the incidence of withdrawal from

Table 4
Variables for 9 neonates born from July 2006–December 2011 in whom NEC developed while in the NICU undergoing treatment for abstinence syndrome associated with maternal opioid narcotic use during pregnancy

Area of State	Birth Wt (g)	Gest Age (w.d)	Gender	Maternal Medications (and/or Illicit Drugs)	Medications Given to Neonate Before NEC	Age when NEC Developed (d)	Feedings Before NEC Diagnosis
South	2740	38.6	M	Suboxone, Tobacco	Amp, Gent	2	Enf 20 (NG+PO)
South	3232	39.2	F	Nubain, Lortab, Zoloft, Prozac, Tobacco	None	2	Breast
SLC	3405	39.5	M	Methadone, Tobacco	Amp, Gent, Morph, Clonidine	8	Enf 20 (NG+PO)
SLC	3015	38.2	F	Methadone, Cocaine	Pheno, Morph	19	Sim 20 (NG+PO)
North	3470	39.6	M	Methadone	Pheno, Morph	9	Sim 20 (NG+PO)
SLC	2730	36.6	M	Methadone, Xanax, Tobacco	Pheno, Morph	20	Enf 20
North	2965	38.1	M	Suboxone	Clonidine, Pheno	5	Enf 20
SLC	2685	39.4	M	Methadone	Pheno	5	Enf 20 (NG+PO)
North	3530	40.2	F	Suboxone, Methadone, Cocaine, Heroin, Ecstasy, Tobacco	Clonidine, Morph	8	Sim 20

Abbreviations: Amp, ampicillin; Enf, Enfamil; Gent, gentamicin; Gest, gestational; Morph, morphine sulfate; NG, nasogastric; Pheno, phenobarbital; PO, per os (oral feeding by nipple); Sim, Similac; SLC, Salt Lake City.

Table 5		
Common features of term neonates in whom NEC develops		
	Feature	**Example**
1	Admitted to an NICU for some reason other than NEC (NEC develops as a complication during the NICU treatment course).	Suspected sepsis, congenital heart disease, polycythemia
2	The underlying medical problem involves compromised gastrointestinal perfusion or function.	Reduced mesenteric perfusion (polycythemia, univentricular heart, sepsis). Withdrawal from maternal opioid narcotics.
3	Feeding plans	Gavage feeding. Cow's milk–based formula. Fed a larger volume than breast feeding neonates would likely receive.

maternal opioid use between 2000 and 2009. They estimated that about 13,500 neonates in the United States annually undergo hospital-managed narcotic withdrawal, many of which stem from chronic pain management of pregnant women.[24,25]

Neonates undergoing opioid withdrawal can be very irritable. This can be misinterpreted as hunger and treated with oral or gavage feedings in excess of physiologic volumes. Because mother's own milk supply can be limited in the first few days, and because some caregivers might advocate not using mother's own milk in which her drug intake is uncertain, cow's milk–based formulas, and overfeeding, are probably fairly common in this population.

Opioid receptors are expressed on cells in the central nervous system, peripheral nervous system, and intestine.[26,27] Withdrawal from chronic opioids typically generates gastrointestinal symptoms, including cramping, bloating, and diarrhea.[28–30] The authors speculate that term NEC among neonates undergoing hospital-managed withdrawal is similar to the other cases of term NEC in the sense that they were admitted to an NICU for a problem involving poor mesenteric perfusion (or other gastrointestinal impairment) then overfed using cow's milk–based formula.[22,31]

In any NICU this new variety of NEC (opioid withdrawal) would likely be too rare to notice. However, using a multicentered database, the emergence of this pattern is clear. We suspect that, although not previously described, this variety might currently constitute one of the most common causes of NEC among term neonates.

Potential ways to reduce term NEC associated with opioid withdrawal include first recognizing that the entity exists, not feeding these patients more than breast-fed neonates of the same age might normally receive,[22] not interpreting their crying and extreme fussiness as hunger, not treating these symptoms with gavage feedings, and using mother's own milk when feasible.[32,33]

SUMMARY

NEC is the most common gastrointestinal emergency of preterm neonates,[1] but since 1973, it has also been known to occur, albeit rarely, among term neonates.[2–18,34–41] Among 52 cases of term NEC during an 11-year period, the authors found no case in which NEC developed in a completely well neonate. Rather, all had some antecedent illness or condition requiring NICU admission (**Table 5**). On this basis, the authors maintain that term NEC develops among those with predispositions. If this is correct, the problem of preventing term NEC may be less daunting than we initially anticipated. Specifically, if term NEC is viewed as a condition occurring in one per 20,000 term neonates, prevention schemes would be exceedingly difficult to test because of the large number needed to treat to prevent one case. However, if term NEC is viewed as a complication arising among a select subset of NICU patients, targeted prevention schemes could be practical.

Conditions that increase the risk of term NEC include congenital heart disease, particularly functionally univentricular heart syndromes, polycythemia, perinatal asphyxia, hypotension including early-onset bacterial infection, and neonatal abstinence from opioid narcotics. The authors suspect that a common feature of these is reduced mesenteric perfusion followed by overfeeding using cow's milk–based formulas. McElhinney and colleagues[11] came to this conclusion when studying term NEC in neonates with congenital heart disease. They reported that patients with shock had the highest odds of NEC development, and they ascribed this association to reduced mesenteric perfusion.

In a neonatal animal model of overfeeding, NEC-like mucosal and submucosal injury occurs.[31] Reports by deGamarra and colleagues,[4] Andrews and colleagues,[7] Martinez-Tallo and colleagues,[8] and Maayan-Metzger and colleagues[15] mentioned that every term neonate in whom NEC developed had been fed before NEC developed. Martinez-Tallo and colleagues[8] and Maayan-Metzger and colleagues[15] reported that all had been fed artificial formula, not breast milk. We reported that most these are overfed.[22] In preterm neonates, a protective effect of human milk toward NEC has been reported.[1] Whether breast feeding protects term neonates from NEC is unproven, but this is consistent with multiple reports.

Successful efforts are needed to prevent NEC among term neonates. It seems to us that such efforts can focus on term neonates admitted to an NICU in which the pathophysiology involves reduced mesenteric perfusion or withdrawal from opioid narcotics. Perhaps reasonable starting places for prevention trials among such neonates could include human milk feeding programs and avoidance of overfeeding, particularly gavage feedings.

REFERENCES

1. Neu J, Mihatsch W. Recent developments in necrotizing enterocolitis. JPEN J Parenter Enteral Nutr 2012;36(Suppl):30–5.
2. Rodin AE, Nichols NM, Hsu FL. Necrotizing enterocolitis occurring in full-term neonates at birth. Arch Pathol 1973;96:335–8.
3. Polin RA, Pollack PF, Barlow B, et al. Necrotizing enterocolitis in term infants. J Pediatr 1976;89:460–2.
4. deGamarra E, Helardot P, Moriette G, et al. Necrotizing enterocolitis in full-term newborns. Biol Neonate 1983;44:185–92.
5. Goldbert RN, Thomas DW, Sinatra FR. Necrotizing enterocolitis in the asphyxiated full-term infant. Am J Perinatol 1983;1:40–2.
6. Thilo EH, Lazarte RA, Hernandez JA. Necrotizing enterocolitis in the first 24 hours of life. Pediatrics 1984;73:476–80.
7. Andrews DA, Sawin RS, Ledbetter DJ, et al. Necrotizing enterocolitis in term neonates. Am J Surg 1990;159:507–9.
8. Martinez-Tallo E, Claure N, Bancalari E. Necrotizing enterocolitis in full-term or near-term infants: risk factors. Biol Neonate 1997;71:292–8.
9. Fatica C, Gordon S, Mossad E, et al. A cluster of necrotizing enterocolitis in term infants undergoing open-heart surgery. Am J Infect Control 2000;28: 130–2.

10. Bolisetty S, Lui KJ, Oei J, et al. A regional study of underlying congenital diseases in term neonates with necrotizing enterocolitis. Acta Paediatr 2000;89:1226–30.

11. McElhinney DB, Hedrick HL, Bush DM, et al. Necrotizing enterocolitis in neonates with congenital heart disease: risk factors and outcomes. Pediatrics 2000;106: 1080–7.

12. Buangtrakool R, Laohapensang M, Sathornkich C, et al. Necrotizing enterocolitis: a comparison between full-term and pre-term neonates. J Med Assoc Thai 2001; 84:323–31.

13. Ng S. Necrotizing enterocolitis in the full-term neonate. J Paediatr Child Health 2001;37:1–4.

14. Ostlie DJ, Spilde TL, St Peter SD, et al. Necrotizing enterocolitis in full-term infants. J Pediatr Surg 2003;38:1039–42.

15. Maayan-Metzger A, Itzchak A, Mazkereth R, et al. Necrotizing enterocolitis in full-term infants: case-control study and review of the literature. J Perinatol 2004;24:494–9.

16. Siahanidou T, Mandyla H, Anagnostakis D, et al. Twenty-six full-term neonates with necrotizing enterocolitis. J Pediatr Surg 2004;39:79.

17. Lambert DK, Christensen RD, Henry E, et al. Necrotizing enterocolitis in term neonates: data from a multihospital health-care system. J Perinatol 2007;27(7): 437–43.

18. Gordon PV. The little database that could: Intermountain Health Care and the uphill quest for prevention of term necrotizing enterocolitis. J Perinatol 2007; 27(7):397–8.

19. Bell MJ, Shackelford P, Feigin RD, et al. Epidemiologic and bacteriologic evaluation of neonatal necrotizing enterocolitis. J Pediatr Surg 1997;14:1–4.

20. Walsh MC, Kliegman RM. Necrotizing enterocolitis: treatment based on staging criteria. Pediatr Clin North Am 1986;33:179–202.

21. Vermont Oxford Network Database. Manual of Operations. Release 10.0, 2005. pp 77, 78.

22. Stout G, Lambert DK, Baer VL, et al. Necrotizing enterocolitis during the first week of life: a multicentered case-control and cohort comparison study. J Perinatol 2008;28(8):556–60.

23. Patrick SW, Schumacher RE, Benneyworth BD, et al. Neonatal abstinence syndrome and associated health care expenditures: United States, 2000-2009. JAMA 2012;307(18):1934–40.

24. Buchi KF, Suarez C, Varner MW. The prevalence of prenatal opioid and other drug use in Utah. Am J Perinatol 2012. [Epub ahead of print].

25. Bell SG. Buprenorphine: a newer drug for treating neonatal abstinence syndrome. Neonatal Netw 2012;31(3):178–83.

26. Jansson LM, Velez M. Neonatal abstinence syndrome. Curr Opin Pediatr 2012; 24(2):252–8.

27. Bio LL, Siu A, Poon CY. Update on the pharmacologic management of neonatal abstinence syndrome. J Perinatol 2011;31(11):692–701.

28. Blandthorn J, Forster DA, Love V. Neonatal and maternal outcomes following maternal use of buprenorphine or methadone during pregnancy: findings of a retrospective audit. Women Birth 2011;24(1):32–9.

29. Peng J, Sarkar S, Chang SL. Opioid receptor expression in human brain and peripheral tissues using absolute quantitative real-time RT-PCR. Drug Alcohol Depend 2012;124(3):223–8.

30. Holzer P. Treatment of opioid-induced gut dysfunction. Expert Opin Investig Drugs 2007;16(2):181–94.

31. Okada K, Fujii T, Ohtsuka Y, et al. Overfeeding can cause NEC-like enterocolitis in premature rat pups. Neonatology 2010;97(3):218–24.
32. Isemann B, Meinzen-Derr J, Akinbi H. Maternal and neonatal factors impacting response to methadone therapy in infants treated for neonatal abstinence syndrome. J Perinatol 2011;31(1):25–9.
33. Jansson LM, Choo R, Velez ML, et al. Methadone maintenance and breastfeeding in the neonatal period. Pediatrics 2008;121(1):106–14.
34. Raboei EH. Necrotizing enterocolitis in full-term neonates: is it aganglionosis? Eur J Pediatr Surg 2009;19(2):101–4.
35. Carlo WF, Kimball TR, Michelfelder EC, et al. Persistent diastolic flow reversal in abdominal aortic Doppler-flow profiles is associated with an increased risk of necrotizing enterocolitis in term infants with congenital heart disease. Pediatrics 2007;119(2):330–5.
36. Christensen RD, Lambert DK, Schmutz N, et al. Fatal bowel necrosis in two poly-cytemic term neonates. Fetal Pediatr Pathol 2008;27(1):41–4.
37. van der Meulen EF, Bergman KA, Kamps AW. Necrotising enterocolitis in a term neonate with trisomy 21 exposed to maternal HIV and antiretroviral medication. Eur J Pediatr 2009;168(1):113–4.
38. Cichocki M, Singer G, Beyerlein S, et al. A case of necrotizing enterocolitis associated with adenovirus infection in a term infant with 22q11 deletion syndrome. J Pediatr Surg 2008;43(4):e5–8.
39. Guner YS, Malhotra A, Ford HR, et al. Association of Escherichia coli O157:H7 with necrotizing enterocolitis in a full-term infant. Pediatr Surg Int 2009;25(5):459–63.
40. Gill D. Necrotizing enterocolitis in a 16-day-old, term neonate. Emerg Med Australas 2011;23(4):507–9.
41. Krishnan L, Pathare A. Necrotizing enterocolitis in a term neonate following intravenous immunoglobulin therapy. Indian J Pediatr 2011;78(6):743–4.

Lactoferrin and Necrotizing Enterocolitis

Michael P. Sherman, MD

KEYWORDS

- Lactoferrin • Necrotizing enterocolitis • Prophylaxis • Intelectin • Toll-like receptors
- Endotoxin binding • Dendritic cells • Th1 cells

KEY POINTS

- Lactoferrin (LF) is a multi-functional protein and a member of the transferrin family.
- LF and lysozyme in breast milk kill bacteria. In the stomach, pepsin digests and releases a potent peptide antibiotic called lactoferricin from native LF.
- The antimicrobial characteristics of LF may facilitate a healthy intestinal microbiome.
- The immunomodulatory activates of LF activate dendritic cells and dendritic cells then induce a T-helper type 1 helper cell population that resists neonatal infection.
- LF has anti-inflammatory actions that may mitigate the pro-inflammatory state that is present in the gut before the onset of necrotizing enterocolitis.
- LF is the major whey in human milk; its highest concentration is in colostrum. This fact highlights early feeding of colostrum and also fresh mature milk as a way to prevent necrotizing enterocolitis.

INTRODUCTION

Five years ago the National Institute of Child Health and Human Development published a workshop report discussing new therapies and preventive approaches for necrotizing enterocolitis (NEC).[1] This conference, and a more recent review,[2] emphasized the importance of mother's milk in averting NEC. Several molecules in human milk may interact and provide a substantial benefit in preventing NEC, but the actual mechanisms remain incomplete.[3] Specific prebiotics in human milk likely shape a healthy intestinal microbiota and thus hinder the invasion of epithelia by bacterial pathogens, but a recent review stated prebiotics have no proven effectiveness.[2] Lactoferrin (LF), the major whey protein in human milk,[4] was not

Funding: This work was supported in part by NIH grant HD057744 and a Gerber Foundation grant.
Division of Neonatology, Women's and Children's Hospital, University of Missouri Health System, University of Missouri, Suite 206, 404 Keene Street, Columbia, MO 65201, USA
E-mail address: ShermanMP@health.missouri.edu

mentioned as a protein that might decrease the occurrence of NEC in recent reviews.[1,2] Conversely, reports show that early enteral administration of bovine LF to very low birth weight infants (VLBW; <1500 g birth weight) lowers the incidence of late-onset sepsis (LOS) and NEC.[5] This overview covers (1) a historic perspective of LF as a biologic therapy, (2) the scientific mechanisms whereby LF prevents NEC, (3) preclinical and clinical studies of LF in neonatal animals and man that show efficacy, (4) the current state of clinical trials involving LF that are designed to prevent LOS and NEC, and (5) future directions of research that involve LF and a reduction in NEC.

DISCOVERY OF LACTOFERRIN AS A THERAPEUTIC AGENT

Although identified as a whey protein in 1939, LF was not isolated and purified from human milk until 1960.[4] During the past 50 years, investigations have shown how LF acts in the gastrointestinal tract of neonates to enhance the immune system. The pace of LF-associated research accelerated over the past 20 years because biotechnology made bovine and human LF available for therapeutic applications.[6,7] **Box 1** summarizes the important scientific reports involving LF that are relevant to neonates and the prevention of NEC. This review cites only investigations that ultimately set in motion a clinical trial that used bovine LF prophylactically to treat preterm infants.

In the 1990s, there was evidence LF had significant in vitro antimicrobial activity when lysozyme was present[10] and that the action of pepsin on LF in the stomach released a potent microbicide called lactoferricin (LFcin).[11] After the intake of LF in human milk, the aforesaid events in the stomach probably result in a pathogen-free gastric fluid that enters the duodenum, which is the rationale as to why therapeutic agents that inhibit acid production in neonatal stomach should be used sparingly so pepsin can act on LF to generate LFcin.

In 1998, a well-known formula manufacturer in the United States held the rights to the commercial production of recombinant human lactoferrin (rhLF).[6] The company had no proof that feeding rhLF could prevent an enteric infection in newborn infants. A neonatal animal model was sought by the company that showed prophylaxis with rhLF prevented morbidity and death from bacterial enterocolitis. This neonatal model was reported in 2001.[14] Additional studies using this model led to a clinical trial of bovine LF that showed prophylaxis with LF prevented LOS and NEC in preterm infants.[5] Before addressing preclinical and clinical studies that indicate LF reduces the risk of NEC, it is essential that the multifunctional nature of LF be understood.

BIOCHEMICAL, PHYSIOLOGIC, AND IMMUNOLOGIC CHARACTERISTICS OF LF

LF is a 78-kDa member of the transferrin family and is present in human milk, saliva, tears, airway mucus, and the secondary granules of neutrophils.[4] **Fig. 1** reviews the wide range of actions attributed to LF. The ways that LF prevent NEC include the following: (1) its role in host defense against pathogens,[17,18] (2) its immunomodulatory and anti-inflammatory effects,[13,16,19,20] (3) its regulation of intestinal cell growth,[9,21,22] and (4) its biochemical actions that include ferric iron transport,[23,24] enzymatic activity,[25,26] and nuclear binding and initiation of transcription.[18,27,28]

The pathophysiology of NEC is complex, but several factors are accepted as effectors of the disease.[1,2,29–31] NEC occurs frequently in VLBW infants. Enteral feedings have often been instituted before disease onset. A less diverse intestinal microbiota with pathogenic characteristics is associated with microbial invasion

Box 1		
Lactoferrin-related research leading to its use to prevent necrotizing enterocolitis		
Year	Discovery and Meaning	Citation
1972	Lactoferrin (LF) with low amounts of bound Fe^{3+} iron, called apo-lactoferrin, restricts the growth of *Escherichia coli*. The study proposed LF in breast milk controls the growth of gut-related bacterial pathogens.	[8]
1987	Human LF increased thymidine incorporation into rat crypt cells and suggests a role for LF in intestinal growth after birth.	[9]
1991	LF and lysozyme, antibacterial proteins in milk, have an additive effect and kill enteric pathogens.	[10]
1991	A "nicked" 78-kDa LF that was largely intact was identified in the urine of preterm infants; the modified protein retained iron-binding activity, receptor-binding properties, and the proposed immune cell regulatory functions. The "nicked" protein may represent removal of peptide antibiotics.[11]	[12]
1995	In infant mice, human LF is a maturation factor for B cells enhancing their phenotype and function; this might mediate more secretory IgA into gut lumen.	[13]
1995	Human LF was expressed in *Aspergillus awamori* and a fully functional protein could be produced in large quantities using good manufacturing practices.	[6]
1998	In the stomach, pepsin releases a "defensinlike" peptide from LF that is called lactoferricin, which disrupts cell membranes of gram-negative enteric bacteria.	[11]
2001	Feeding human recombinant LF to neonatal rats before an intestinal infection with *E coli* significantly reduces translocation, bacteremia, and death.	[14]
2004	Feeding recombinant human LF + *Lactobacillus rhamnosus* GG (LGG) had more of an effect than feeding LGG alone in reducing gut-related translocation after an enteral infection with *E coli*; recombinant human LF enhanced intestinal colonization with LGG. This research was the basis for the first clinical trial of LF in preterm infants.	[15]
2005	Feeding LF and vitamin A to calves enhances epithelial cell maturation, villus growth, and size and nature of Peyer's patches. An accelerated development of Peyer's patches may result in increased production of secretory IgA.	[16]
2009	In very preterm infants, oral prophylaxis with bovine LF + LGG significantly reduced late-onset sepsis and necrotizing enterocolitis compared with bovine LF only and placebo. Bovine LF + LGG vs bLF alone had no difference when necrotizing enterocolitis stage ≥ 2 and death were the outcomes ($P = .06$).	[5]

or adverse effects of their toxins on intestinal epithelia. Hence, NEC always associates with inflammation of gut-related tissues. Intestinal inflammation reduces blood flow and is associated with coagulation necrosis of the bowel as the endpoint in NEC.

The lone strategy that decreases the risk of NEC was reported 20 years ago.[32] To ease the occurrence of NEC, exclusive feeding of milk from a preterm infant's mother should be the mainstay of neonatal care for VLBW infants.[33] Nevertheless, many VLBW infants have a low intake of colostrum or milk in the days following birth. The authors' hypothesis stated "feeding of lactoferrin in sufficient amounts from the first day of life may lessen the prevalence of NEC." The following bulleted points present

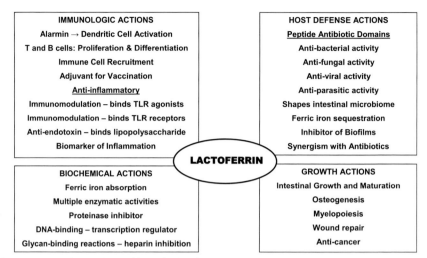

IMMUNOLOGIC ACTIONS	HOST DEFENSE ACTIONS
Alarmin → Dendritic Cell Activation	Peptide Antibiotic Domains
T and B cells: Proliferation & Differentiation	Anti-bacterial activity
Immune Cell Recruitment	Anti-fungal activity
Adjuvant for Vaccination	Anti-viral activity
Anti-inflammatory	Anti-parasitic activity
Immunomodulation – binds TLR agonists	Shapes intestinal microbiome
Immunomodulation – binds TLR receptors	Ferric iron sequestration
Anti-endotoxin – binds lipopolysaccharide	Inhibitor of Biofilms
Biomarker of Inflammation	Synergism with Antibiotics

LACTOFERRIN

BIOCHEMICAL ACTIONS	GROWTH ACTIONS
Ferric iron absorption	Intestinal Growth and Maturation
Multiple enzymatic activities	Osteogenesis
Proteinase inhibitor	Myelopoiesis
DNA-binding – transcription regulator	Wound repair
Glycan-binding reactions – heparin inhibition	Anti-cancer

Fig. 1. Four major actions of lactoferrin that may act to prevent necrotizing enterocolitis.

in greater depth specific actions of LF that are responsible for diminishing the risk of NEC in preterm infants.

- Breast milk contains LF and lysozyme that can act together in the stomach to destroy gram-positive and gram-negative pathogens, and this eliminates their damaging toxins on epithelia or mucosal invasion.[10,14,17]
- Whether breast feeding is or is not being used for nourishment, consuming LF can release LFcin in the stomach. LFcin kills a wide range of bacterial, fungal, viral, and parasitic pathogens.[17,18] Antagonists of acid production in the stomach should be avoided in VLBW infants so pepsin can release LFcin from LF.[20]
- The 2 mechanisms listed above produce a gastric fluid that is free of pathogens. This nearly sterile gastric fluid enters the small intestine. LF is particularly resistant to proteolytic degradation in the alimentary tract compared with other milk proteins like casein.[12,34] Thus, intact LF is still available in the small bowel to act with lysozyme or other peptide antibiotics (eg, defensins) secreted by Paneth cells; together they can damage or kill microbes.[35,36] LFcin also acts within the lumen of the small intestine.[17,18]
- LF has several other actions in which it participates within the lumen of the small bowel. LF can still block toxicity to or invasion of epithelia by microorganisms. This mechanism avoids epithelia-related injury and involves LF binding to microbial molecules (eg, endotoxin, CpG, peptidoglycan), bacterial flagellin (disrupts motility), or cellular determinants that pathogens use for adherence (eg, CD14, Toll-like receptors: -2, -4, -5, and -9).[20,35,37] These actions are vital to host defense against pathogens, but the effect is also anti-inflammatory (**Fig. 2**). This latter consequence of LF prophylaxis is fundamental to decreasing the inflammation associated with NEC in preterm infants.
- LF may provide an initial level of protection via its glycan chains that contain sialic acid, which bind proteins of viruses and bacteria.[38] Binding of viruses or bacteria to the glycan moiety of LF means pathogens can be carried from the body on LF and eliminated in the feces.

A second mechanism also eliminates bacteria that invade enterocytes. When neonatal rats were pretreated with rhLF and then infected with enteral *Escherichia*

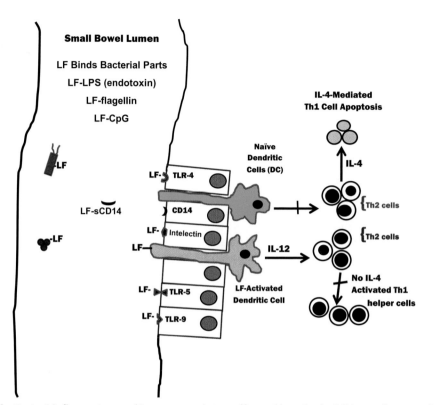

Fig. 2. Anti-inflammatory and immunoregulatory effects of lactoferrin (LF) in small neonatal intestine. LF binds several bacterial components including cell wall–associated lipopolysaccharide (LPS), flagellin, and DNA (CpG). This binding inhibits the bacterial components from initiating an inflammatory response. LF also binds to gram-positive or gram-negative bacteria either killing the microbe or hindering its invasion of tissue. LF engages pattern recognition receptors (ie, Toll-like receptors [TLR], CD14 receptor) on gut-related epithelia and thereby restricts transduction of a pro-inflammatory signal or microbial translocation. By adhering to its own receptor, the lipid raft intelectin, LF further limits infection. Importantly, LF activates dendritic cells (DCs) as they provide surveillance of the gut lumen. This LF-initiated signaling mediates secretion of intereukin-12 (IL-12) by DCs, which in turn stops interleukin-4 (IL-4) production by T-helper type 2 (Th2) cells and reverses apoptotic death of T-helper type 1 (Th1) cells. This process creates a competent Th1 helper cell population and restores a proper Th1/Th2 balance that can resist infection.

coli, a phenomenon called anoikis was observed.[39] Apoptotic epithelia were shed from the mucosa surface, and they contained intracellular *E coli*. This mechanism is a way to rid the mucosa of infected cells; the apoptotic enterocytes with trapped bacteria inside are released into the lumen and leave the body via peristalsis. This process was not seen in infected neonatal rats that were treated with placebo rather than rhLF.

- The protease activity of LF is used to degrade secreted bacterial proteins that are used by enteric pathogens to form a needle and create pores in host epithelia.[40] This mechanism of bacterial invasion applies to several enteric microbes. In addition, serine protease activity of LF cleaves surface proteins at arginine-rich sites of *Haemophilus influenzae* and interferes with their viability.[41] This microbicidal mechanism is applicable to bacterial pathogens other than *Haemophilus*.

- Iron sequestration mediated by LF was reported by Bullen and colleagues[8] in 1972. This aspect of ferric ion metabolism is no longer considered a major antibacterial mechanism in the intestinal lumen. However, LF-mediated iron sequestration in the lung causes twitching motility in *Pseudomonas aeruginosa* and this prevents the bacterium from forming biofilms.[42] Proof exists that biofilm formation occurs on the intestinal mucosa,[43,44] but the role of LF in its prevention has not been studied.
- The proliferation and differentiation of intestinal epithelia are stimulated by LF.[9,21,22,45] LF is absorbed from the intestine by means of a specific receptor, Intelectin, that is located on brush border cells.[46–48] The binding to LF to intelectin hinders pathogens from adhering to lipid rafts and thereby gaining entry into epithelia.[48] LF also plays a role in the absorption of nutrients.[7,22,49] The protein can deliver such metal ions as iron, manganese, and zinc and facilitate the absorption of sugars. Whether treatment with LF renders these epithelia less susceptible to toxins or microbial invasion remains to be investigated. Whether tight junctions are more competent after exposure to LF also needs to be studied. Last, LF added to formula increased hepatic protein synthesis akin to piglets given colostrum, and this finding has implications for host defense.[50]

The preceding bullet points addressed the actions of LF related to intestinal host defenses and how these mechanisms reduce gut-related inflammation and infection. The bullet points that follow outline how LF acts on a nascent immune system in the intestine.

- Neonatal studies addressing the influence of LF on T- and B-cell physiology are limited. Adult studies show that LF induces immature T-cell precursors to differentiate via the CD4 antigen.[51] When LF binds with monophoshoryl lipid A, an endotoxin component, it acts as an efficient adjuvant of the humoral and cellular immune responses.[52] This observation is important because LF may alter the T-helper type 1/T-helper type 2 (Th2/Th1) bias of neonates that is associated with an increased risk of infections.[53]
- Phenotypic changes are induced when splenic B cells of mice are treated with human LF; this treatment also increases surface IgD and complement receptor expression.[13] Human LF enabled B cells from normal newborn and adult immunodeficient CBA/N mice to present antigen to an antigen-specific Th2 cell line.[13]
- LF given orally to calves increases the size of Peyer's patches in the ileum and blood levels of immunoglobulin G.[16] Neonatal rats fed rhLF and *Lactobacillus rhamnosus* GG (LGG) compared with LGG alone had an accelerated appearance of "domed villi," the precursors of Peyer's patches.[15] This finding may result in increased IgA secretion into the intestinal lumen.[54]
- This point is the most important of the review. A human recombinant LF, designated talactoferrin (TLF), acts as an alarmin and promotes the recruitment and activation of antigen-presenting cells.[55] Immunization of mice with ovalbumin in the presence of TLF promoted Th1-polarized antigen-specific immune responses. TLF is also a novel maturation factor for monocyte conversion to dendritic cells.[56] TLF increases the capacity of dendritic cells to trigger proliferation and release interferon-γ in the presence of allogeneic human T cells. It is proposed that LF-mediated maturation of dendritic cells allows secretion of interleukin (IL)-12.[20] In turn, IL-12 stops Th2-associated production of IL-4, saving Th1 cells from IL-4-mediated apoptosis (see **Fig. 2**). This mechanism overcomes a neonatal bias for Th2 cells over Th1 cells; Th2 bias makes infants susceptible to infections.[57] TLF-mediated enhancement of Th1 numbers and functions was

likely responsible for the benefit observed during neonatal studies that used TLF prophylaxis to improve outcomes after enteral infection with E coli.[14,15] How these studies lead to a clinical trial that did reduce NEC are discussed later.

STUDIES OF LACTOFERRIN TO PREVENT NEONATAL INFECTIONS
Preclinical Studies

Neonatal animal models of NEC have not been used to evaluate whether LF can either mitigate the disease process or reduce it altogether. Two studies have used prophylaxis with rhLF (ie, TLF) to reduce bacterial translocation after enteral infection with E coli.

The initial study used neonatal rats and administered rhLF at a dose similar to human breast-fed infants.[14] Rat milk has miniscule amounts of LF.[58] Treated pups received 2 days of rhLF before being infected with intragastric E coli on successive days. The prophylaxis had the 4 following beneficial effects: (1) a 3 log reduction in colony forming units of E coli in the blood ($P<.001$), (2) 50% lower colony forming units of E coli in liver cultures ($P<.02$), (3) a marked reduction in illness scores in the surviving pups ($P<.001$), and (4) a 8% mortality in treated pups versus 57% mortality in rats given placebo ($P<.001$). Histologic studies showed a marked reduction in villus-related pathologic abnormality in infected pups given prophylactic LF compared with the controls. No gross or microscopic findings of NEC were observed in either treated or control groups.

A second study was designed differently. It was hypothesized that rhLF would facilitate colonization of small bowel with LGG. It was proposed that rhLF + LGG would prevent bacterial translocation more effectively compared with LGG alone. Bacterial translocation was measured after enteral infection with E coli by culturing the luminal fluid followed by enumeration of colony forming units of E coli in the homogenized bowel wall. Control pups had lactic acid bacteria in the bowel, but they were not LGG. Pups treated with LGG or rhLF + LGG had significantly higher numbers of LGG in the ileum versus jejunum. Contrary to the hypothesis, rhLF did not augment LGG colonization. After gut infection, E coli in bowel lumen and E coli adherent to epithelia and invading the bowel wall were reduced by pretreatment with rhLF and LGG ($P<.05$). These 2 preclinical studies resulted in a randomized clinic trial (RCT) that fed bovine LF (bLF) or bLF + LGG to prevent infection in VLBW infants.

Clinical Studies

Only 1 RCT that has used prophylactic LF in preterm infants has been published to date.[5,59] The primary outcome was a reduction in LOS caused by bacteria or fungi. The occurrence of stage 2 or stage 3 NEC was a secondary outcome. The study used bLF or bLF + LGG as a preventive strategy. A single daily dose of 30 to −150 mg bLF was used in the first 2 weeks. The infants weighing less than 1000 g at birth were treated for 6 weeks and infants weighing less than 1500 g at birth were treated for 4 weeks. The incidence of LOS was 17.3% in the control group (n = 168), whereas the incidence of LOS was 5.9% in the bLF group (n = 153, $P = .002$) and 4.6% in the bLF + LGG group (n = 151, $P<.001$), respectively. If infants with birth weights of 1000 to 1500 g are examined separately, there was not a significant reduction in LOS (bLF, $P = .34$ and bLF + LGG, $P = .07$). Death from sepsis was significantly lower in infants with birth weights less than 1500 g if they received prophylaxis with bLF or bLF + LGG. Infants fed maternal milk exclusively had an additive effect on reducing infection, which was a confounding variable.

Stage 2 to stage 3 NEC was reduced in the bLF + LGG group (0/151, P = .002) compared with the bLF group (3/153, P = .09) and control (10/168). This report has been accepted by neonatologists with much enthusiasm, but it must be considered preliminary. Because of the low risk of NEC in very preterm infants, confirmatory studies that use LF to prevent NEC must be performed with a large enough sample size.

CURRENT STATE OF NEONATAL CLINICAL TRIALS USING LACTOFERRIN

In reviewing the roster of research projects at ClinicalTrials.gov, there is no single-centered or multicentered RCT that uses LF exclusively to prevent NEC. **Box 2**

Box 2
Neonatal studies of lactoferrin to reduce necrotizing enterocolitis and listed in ClinicalTrials.gov

Title, Institution, and Location	Agent/Dose	Primary Outcome	Type of Patients and Number of Subjects	Status
Pilot Study: Lactoferrin for Prevention of Neonatal Sepsis (NEOLACTO) Universidad Peruana Cayetano Heredia, Lima, Peru	Bovine LF; 200 mg/kg/d divided into 3 doses/d for 4 wk	Late-onset sepsis (LOS)	Infants: <2500 g birth weight; N = 190, extended to 414 newborns	Closed, abstract[60]
Study of Talactoferrin Oral Solution for Nosocomial Infection in Preterm Infants University of Missouri, USA University of Louisville, USA University of Southern California, USA	Human recombinant lactoferrin; 150 mg/dose twice daily, 4 wk	LOS	Infants: 750–1500 g birth weight; N = 120 (phase I and II)	Closed, in data analyses
Oral Lactoferrin Prophylaxis to Prevent Sepsis and Necrotizing Enterocolitis of Very Low Birth Weight Neonates in Neonatal Intensive Care Unit and Effect on T-regulatory Cells Ankara University, Turkey	Bovine LF; 200 mg/d, given with either human milk or preterm formula	LOS and NEC	Infants: <1500 g birth weight and <32 wk gestation; N = 60	Recruiting

summarizes the completed or ongoing studies that use LF to prevent LOS and are not yet published.

The Peruvian study reported its results at the 2012 Pediatric Academic Society meeting.[60] Enrollment included 190 infants weighing less than 2500 g at birth. bLF (Tatua, Morrinsville, New Zealand) and placebo (maltodextrin) were given enterally at 200 mg/d in 3 divided doses over the first 4 weeks of life. Nutrition consisted of maternal milk in 67% of infants and 32% of the premature infants received formula. The cumulative incidence of sepsis in the bLF group was 12/95 (12.6%) compared with 22/95 (23.2%) in the placebo group. For infants weighing less than 1500 g at birth, the occurrence of NEC was 20% in the bLF group (8/40) versus 40% in the control group (16/40). The study did not have statistical significance, but the reduction of NEC in the LF group was approximately 50%. No data were provided about the occurrence of NEC. There were no adverse events in infants that received enteral bLF. This study is now extended to 414 subjects.

Multicentered studies of LF to prevent NEC are needed and those investigations must be sufficiently powered to achieve an answer about its effectiveness in preterm infants weighing less than 1000 g and 1000 to 1500 g at birth.

FUTURE DIRECTIONS INVOLVING LACTOFERRIN AND REDUCTION OF NEC

There are several challenges for investigators who wish to pursue the efficacy of LF in preventing or mitigating NEC. The following bullet points state those concerns.

- A product that can achieve licensing is needed. Only TLF has Investigational New Drug status from the Food and Drug Administration (FDA). bLF does not have Investigational New Drug status. TLF has been tested extensively in vitro and in vivo for genotoxic effects, mutagenicity, dose ranging toxicity studies in animals and man, sterility and stability, pharmacokinetics, presence of endotoxin or infectious agents, and information on the formation of antibodies after oral administration. A company applying for drug licensure has to prove it is made using Good Manufacturing Practices.
- Two different bLF products have been used in 2 RCTs. The bLF used in the report by Manzoni and coworkers[5] from Italy was a biologic agent made at Dicofarm SpA (Rome, Italy), whereas the study by Ochoa and colleagues from Peru used bLF obtained from Tatua Co-operative Dairy Company (Morrinsville, New Zealand).[60] These preparations are food additives and the FDA designates them as Generally Regarded As Safe. Thus, the standard is high for licensing of a Generally Regarded As Safe product that claims reduction in a major illness. Biologic agents, like humanized monoclonal antibodies that reduce or cure a disease, are usually FDA-approved drugs. For example, probiotic bacteria used to prevent NEC are undergoing substantial scrutiny by the FDA. LF used to prevent LOS or NEC should be a well-characterized biologic agent that passes FDA requirements. An extra criterion that may be required by the FDA is evidence that bLF does not cause bovine spongiform encephalopathy and variant Creutzfeldt-Jakob disease. Thus, LF prophylaxis to prevent NEC may be years away because licensing a biologic agent is rigorous.

SUMMARY

LF-related prophylaxis fulfills an immunologic void if a preterm infant is not taking mother's milk. Scientific evidence is strong that LF enhances immunity in neonates, but only 1 study suggests bovine LF can reduce NEC. LF use in the neonatal intensive care unit to prevent NEC remains problematic because a product must be licensed by the FDA. Given the "state of the art," it is recommended that preterm infants receive colostrum immediately after its collection from the first day of life. Colostrum should be continued until mature milk is available. Mature milk should also be used several times per day right after it has been freshly expressed by the mother. This warning is because freezing or pasteurization significantly lowers the content of LF in the nutrients.[61] Caregivers hope that LF prophylaxis becomes available soon.

REFERENCES

1. Grave GD, Nelson SA, Walker WA, et al. New therapies and preventive approaches for necrotizing enterocolitis: report of a research planning workshop. Pediatr Res 2007;62(4):510–4.
2. Neu J, Walker WA. Necrotizing enterocolitis. N Engl J Med 2011;364(3):255–64.
3. Goldman AS. The immune system in human milk and the developing infant. Breastfeed Med 2007;2(4):195–204.
4. Levay PF, Viljoen M. Lactoferrin: a general review. Haematologica 1995;80(3): 252–67.
5. Manzoni P, Rinaldi M, Cattani S, et al. Bovine lactoferrin supplementation for prevention of late-onset sepsis in very low-birth-weight neonates: a randomized trial. JAMA 2009;302(13):1421–8.
6. Ward PP, Piddington CS, Cunningham GA, et al. A system for production of commercial quantities of human lactoferrin: a broad spectrum natural antibiotic. Biotechnology (NY) 1995;13(5):498–503.
7. Lönnerdal B. Nutritional roles of lactoferrin. Curr Opin Clin Nutr Metab Care 2009; 12(3):293–7.
8. Bullen JJ, Rogers HJ, Leigh L. Iron-binding proteins in milk and resistance to Escherichia coli infection in infants. Br Med J 1972;1(5792):69–75.
9. Nichols BL, McKee KS, Henry JF, et al. Human lactoferrin stimulates thymidine incorporation into DNA of rat crypt cells. Pediatr Res 1987;21(6):563–7.
10. Ellison RT 3rd, Giehl TJ. Killing of gram-negative bacteria by lactoferrin and lysozyme. J Clin Invest 1991;88(4):1080–91.
11. Kuwata H, Yip TT, Tomita M, et al. Direct evidence of the generation in human stomach of an antimicrobial peptide domain (lactoferricin) from ingested lactoferrin. Biochim Biophys Acta 1998;1429(1):129–41.
12. Hutchens TW, Henry JF, Yip TT. Structurally intact (78-kDa) forms of maternal lactoferrin purified from urine of preterm infants fed human milk: identification of a trypsin-like proteolytic cleavage event in vivo that does not result in fragment dissociation. Proc Natl Acad Sci U S A 1991;88(8):2994–8.
13. Zimecki M, Mazurier J, Spik G, et al. Human lactoferrin induces phenotypic and functional changes in murine splenic B cells. Immunology 1995;86(1):122–7.
14. Edde L, Hipolito RB, Hwang FF, et al. Lactoferrin protects neonatal rats from gut-related systemic infection. Am J Physiol Gastrointest Liver Physiol 2001;281(5): G1140–50.
15. Sherman MP, Bennett SH, Hwang FF, et al. Neonatal small bowel epithelia: enhancing anti-bacterial defense with lactoferrin and Lactobacillus GG. Biometals 2004;17(3):285–9.
16. Prgomet C, Prenner ML, Schwarz FJ, et al. Effect of lactoferrin on selected immune system parameters and the gastrointestinal morphology in growing calves. J Anim Physiol Anim Nutr (Berl) 2007;91(3–4):109–19.

17. González-Chávez SA, Arévalo-Gallegos S, Rascón-Cruz Q. Lactoferrin: structure, function and applications. Int J Antimicrob Agents 2009;33(4):301.e1–8.
18. Vogel HJ. Lactoferrin, a bird's eye view. Biochem Cell Biol 2012;90(3):233–44.
19. Legrand D, Mazurier J. A critical review of the roles of host lactoferrin in immunity. Biometals 2010;23(3):365–76.
20. Sherman MP, Adamkin DH, Radmacher PG, et al. Protective proteins in mammalian milks: lactoferrin steps forward. Neoreviews 2012;13(5):e293–300.
21. Buccigrossi V, de Marco G, Bruzzese E, et al. Lactoferrin induces concentration-dependent functional modulation of intestinal proliferation and differentiation. Pediatr Res 2007;61(4):410–4.
22. Liao Y, Jiang R, Lönnerdal B. Biochemical and molecular impacts of lactoferrin on small intestinal growth and development during early life. Biochem Cell Biol 2012; 90(3):476–84.
23. Lopez V, Suzuki YA, Lönnerdal B. Ontogenic changes in lactoferrin receptor and DMT1 in mouse small intestine: implications for iron absorption during early life. Biochem Cell Biol 2006;84(3):337–44.
24. Johnson EE, Wessling-Resnick M. Iron metabolism and the innate immune response to infection. Microbes Infect 2012;14(3):207–16.
25. Furmanski P, Li ZP, Fortuna MB, et al. Multiple molecular forms of human lactoferrin. Identification of a class of lactoferrins that possess ribonuclease activity and lack iron-binding capacity. J Exp Med 1989;170(2):415–29.
26. Kanyshkova TG, Babina SE, Semenov DV, et al. Multiple enzymatic activities of human milk lactoferrin. Eur J Biochem 2003;270(16):3353–61.
27. Fleet JC. A new role for lactoferrin: DNA binding and transcription activation. Nutr Rev 1995;53(8):226–7.
28. Mariller C, Hardivillé S, Hoedt E, et al. Delta-lactoferrin, an intracellular lactoferrin isoform that acts as a transcription factor. Biochem Cell Biol 2012;90(3):307–19.
29. McElroy SJ, Weitkamp JH. Innate immunity in the small intestine of the preterm infant. Neoreviews 2011;12(9):e517–26.
30. Dominguez KM, Moss RL. Necrotizing enterocolitis. Clin Perinatol 2012;39(2): 387–401.
31. McElroy SJ, Underwood MA, Sherman MP. Paneth cells and necrotizing enterocolitis: a novel hypothesis for disease pathogenesis. Neonatology 2012;103(1): 10–20.
32. Lucas A, Cole TJ. Breast milk and neonatal necrotising enterocolitis. Lancet 1990; 336(8730):1519–23.
33. Sullivan S, Schanler RJ, Kim JH, et al. An exclusively human milk-based diet is associated with a lower rate of necrotizing enterocolitis than a diet of human milk and bovine milk-based products. J Pediatr 2010;156(4):562–567.e1.
34. Kuwata H, Yamauchi K, Teraguchi S, et al. Functional fragments of ingested lactoferrin are resistant to proteolytic degradation in the gastrointestinal tract of adult rats. J Nutr 2001;131(8):2121–7.
35. Sherman MP. New concepts of microbial translocation in the neonatal intestine: mechanisms and prevention. Clin Perinatol 2010;37(3):565–79.
36. Bevins CL, Salzman NH. Paneth cells, antimicrobial peptides and maintenance of intestinal homeostasis. Nat Rev Microbiol 2011;9(5):356–68.
37. de Araújo AN, Giugliano LG. Lactoferrin and free secretory component of human milk inhibit the adhesion of enteropathogenic Escherichia coli to HeLa cells. BMC Microbiol 2001;1:25.
38. Baker HM, Baker EN. A structural perspective on lactoferrin function. Biochem Cell Biol 2012;90(3):320–8.

39. Sherman MP, Petrak K. Lactoferrin-enhanced anoikis: a defense against neonatal necrotizing enterocolitis. Med Hypotheses 2005;65(3):478–82.

40. Ochoa TJ, Noguera-Obenza M, Ebel F, et al. Lactoferrin impairs type III secretory system function in enteropathogenic Escherichia coli. Infect Immun 2003;71(9): 5149–55.

41. Hendrixson DR, Qiu J, Shewry SC, et al. Human milk lactoferrin is a serine protease that cleaves Haemophilus surface proteins at arginine-rich sites. Mol Microbiol 2003;47(3):607–17.

42. Singh PK, Parsek MR, Greenberg EP, et al. A component of innate immunity prevents bacterial biofilm development. Nature 2002;417(6888):552–5.

43. Martinez-Medina M, Naves P, Blanco J, et al. Biofilm formation as a novel phenotypic feature of adherent-invasive Escherichia coli (AIEC). BMC Microbiol 2009; 9:202.

44. Macfarlane S, Bahrami B, Macfarlane GT. Mucosal biofilm communities in the human intestinal tract. Adv Appl Microbiol 2011;75:111–43.

45. Lönnerdal B, Jiang R, Du X. Bovine lactoferrin can be taken up by the human intestinal lactoferrin receptor and exert bioactivities. J Pediatr Gastroenterol Nutr 2011;53(6):606–14.

46. Shin K, Wakabayashi H, Yamauchi K, et al. Recombinant human intelectin binds bovine lactoferrin and its peptides. Biol Pharm Bull 2008;31(8):1605–8.

47. Suzuki YA, Wong H, Ashida KY, et al. The N1 domain of human lactoferrin is required for internalization by caco-2 cells and targeting to the nucleus. Biochemistry 2008;47(41):10915–20.

48. Danielsen EM, Hansen GH. Lipid raft organization and function in the small intestinal brush border. J Physiol Biochem 2008;64(4):377–82.

49. Lönnerdal B. Effects of milk and milk components on calcium, magnesium, and trace element absorption during infancy. Physiol Rev 1997;77(3):643–69.

50. Burrin DG, Wang H, Heath J, et al. Orally administered lactoferrin increases hepatic protein synthesis in formula-fed newborn pigs. Pediatr Res 1996;40(1): 72–6.

51. Fischer R, Debbabi H, Dubarry M, et al. Regulation of physiological and pathological Th1 and Th2 responses by lactoferrin. Biochem Cell Biol 2006;84(3): 303–11.

52. Chodaczek G, Zimecki M, Lukasiewicz J, et al. A complex of lactoferrin with monophosphoryl lipid A is an efficient adjuvant of the humoral and cellular immune response in mice. Med Microbiol Immunol 2006;195:207–16.

53. Lee HH, Hoeman CM, Hardaway JC, et al. Delayed maturation of an IL-12-producing dendritic cell subset explains the early Th2 bias in neonatal immunity. J Exp Med 2008;205(10):2269–80.

54. de Moreno de LeBlanc A, Dogi CA, Galdeano CM, et al. Effect of the administration of a fermented milk containing Lactobacillus casei DN-114001 on intestinal microbiota and gut associated immune cells of nursing mice and after weaning until immune maturity. BMC Immunol 2008;9:27.

55. de la Rosa G, Yang D, Tewary P, et al. Lactoferrin acts as an alarmin to promote the recruitment and activation of APCs and antigen-specific immune responses. J Immunol 2008;180(10):6868–76.

56. Spadaro M, Caorsi C, Ceruti P, et al. Lactoferrin, a major defense protein of innate immunity, is a novel maturation factor for human dendritic cells. FASEB J 2008; 22(8):2747–57.

57. Zaghouani H, Hoeman CM, Adkins B. Neonatal immunity: faulty T-helpers and the shortcomings of dendritic cells. Trends Immunol 2009;30(12):585–91.

58. Masson PL, Heremans JF. Lactoferrin in milk from different species. Comp Biochem Physiol B 1971;39(1):119–29.

59. Manzoni P, Stolfi I, Messner H, et al. Bovine lactoferrin prevents invasive fungal infections in very low birth weight infants: a randomized controlled trial. Pediatrics 2012;129(1):116–23.

60. Ochoa TJ, Cam L, Lianos R, et al. Lactoferrin for prevention of sepsis in Peruvian neonates. Abstract from the Proceedings of Pediatric Academic Societies Meeting in Boston, MA, USA, 2012. Pediatric Academic Societies web site, 2012 Abstracts2View, E-PAS2012:2170.7.

61. Evans TJ, Ryley HC, Neale LM, et al. Effect of storage and heat on antimicrobial proteins in human milk. Arch Dis Child 1978;53(3):239–41.

The Altered Gut Microbiome and Necrotizing Enterocolitis

Roberto Murgas Torrazza, MD, Josef Neu, MD*

KEYWORDS

- Necrotizing enterocolitis • Microbiome • Intestinal microbiota
- Noncultured based techniques • Sequencing

KEY POINTS

- The intestinal microbiota normally exist in a commensal or symbiotic relationship with the host, but in the neonate, and especially in the premature infant, this relationship needs to develop.
- Alterations of the intestinal microbiota may predispose the preterm infant to the development of necrotizing enterocolitis.
- Composition and quality of the intestinal microbiota depend on many factors, such as mode of birth, type of feeding, and use of antibiotics. There are many opportunities for physicians to provide interventions that could improve the adequate colonization of the neonatal gut.
- Culture-based techniques are highly limited, but the development of new molecular technologies to study previously unidentified organisms has enhanced our understanding of the microbial environment that may predispose to necrotizing enterocolitis.

INTRODUCTION

Necrotizing enterocolitis (NEC) is an enigmatic disease that has been recognized for more than a century, but with the advent of neonatal intensive care, it has become one of the most common and devastating diseases in neonates.[1–3] Among the reasons why NEC has been so difficult to understand and eradicate is that what has been termed NEC is certainly more than 1 disease with multiple causes.[2] For example, when an infant born at term who has a hypoplastic left ventricle presents with pneumatosis intestinalis at 2 days of age, the cause and pathophysiology of this baby's NEC is likely different from the 25-week gestation preterm who presents with pneumatosis intestinalis at 5 weeks of age. The first is more likely related to ischemic injury caused by hemodynamic insufficiency and hypoxic-ischemic injury[4] rather than

Division of Neonatology, Department of Pediatrics, University of Florida College of Medicine, 1600 Southwest Archer Road, Box 100296, HD Building Room 112, Gainesville, FL 32610-0296, USA
* Corresponding author.
E-mail address: neuj@peds.ufl.edu

Clin Perinatol 40 (2013) 93–108
http://dx.doi.org/10.1016/j.clp.2012.12.009   perinatology.theclinics.com
0095-5108/13/$ – see front matter © 2013 Elsevier Inc. All rights reserved.

a coalescence of factors that result in intestinal inflammation and injury largely as a result of intestinal immaturity, as in the preterm infant. In the latter case, sometimes referred to as classic NEC,[2] the interactions of a predisposing genetic background, an immature intestinal barrier, and a microbial environment that is conducive to the development of NEC are believed to play an interactive and critical role in pathogenesis.[2,3,5]

The linkage of NEC to bacterial colonization was recognized by Santulli and colleagues[6] more than 3 decades ago. Additional observations showing clusters of cases, outbreaks in institutions, the finding of pneumatosis intestinalis, which likely represents submucosal gas produced by bacterial fermentation, and the common findings of bacteremia and endotoxinemia in affected neonates support a microbial role in the pathogenesis of this disease.[5] Numerous bacteria have been related to NEC, but none of them has been found to fulfill Koch's postulates, because they are commonly found among patients without NEC.[7] Viruses have also been implicated in the pathogenesis of NEC, and coronavirus within fecal samples and resected intestinal segments were reported in patients with NEC,[8] but their role in the causation of the disease has not been substantiated.

Recently, the Human Microbiome Project has enabled development of novel technologies that should be highly instrumental in helping understand the contribution of the intestinal microbial ecology to the pathogenesis of NEC.[9] The realization that culture-based techniques are limited in delineating the vast array of microbes present in the human intestine along with the development of new technologies to study these previously unidentified organisms has enhanced our optimism for better describing the microbial environment that may predispose to classic NEC. Furthermore, an appreciation of the role of commensal microbes in protection of the intestine and the disease that may occur when the balance of these commensals is disrupted is opening a new era of thought in the understanding of NEC as well as diseases ranging from obesity to autism. Efforts by the National Institutes of Child Health and Human Development have also paved the way for new studies in NEC.[10] This review focuses on the role of the intestinal microbiota in the pathogenesis of classic NEC.

COMPLEMENTING TRADITIONAL CULTURE-BASED TECHNIQUES

The traditional view of the human is that they are composed of 10 trillion cells, which are the product of approximately 23,000 genes. However, in various niches of the human body, there reside several species of microbes and microbial genes that vastly outnumber those of the human host. In the past few years, emerging technologies derived largely from the Human Genome Project have been applied to evaluating the intestinal microbiota, and new discoveries using these techniques have prompted new initiatives such as the Human Microbiome Roadmap, designed to evaluate the role of the intestinal microbiome in health and disease.

Until the beginning of the last decade, culture-based techniques were the mainstay of evaluating intestinal microbes. However, most bacterial cells seen microscopically in feces cannot be cultured in the laboratory (**Fig. 1**).[11] Recently developed high-throughput molecular techniques analyze microbial DNA and RNA. There are 2 general approaches, both of which comprise several variants. One commonly used general approach is to use the 16S rRNA gene[12] and the other is a more complex metagenomic approach, in which community DNA is subject to shotgun (whole-genome) sequencing.[13] A comprehensive review of these techniques is beyond the scope of this article, but some of the more commonly used techniques are summarized in **Box 1**.

Both methods include the extraction of community DNA or RNA from feces or other samples of interest. The 16S rRNA is a part of the ribosomal RNA. It is commonly used

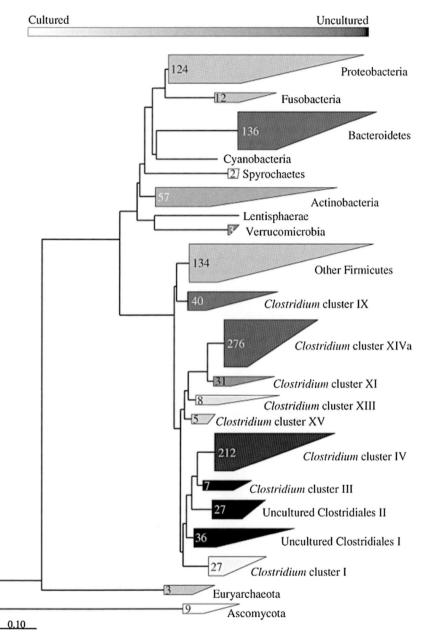

Cultured   Uncultured

Fig. 1. Intestinal microbiota remain mostly uncultured by traditional culture-based methods. Black fills indicate phylotypes detected in cultivation-independent studies and white indicates species detected in cultivation-based studies. (*From* Rajilic-Stojanovic M, Smidt H, de Vos WM. Diversity of the human gastrointestinal tract microbiota revisited. Environ Microbiol 2007;9:2125–36; with permission.)

Box 1

Nonculture techniques of intestinal microbiota identification

16s rRNA sequencing V3/V4 and V4/V5 regions

Shotgun approach: Illumina (Illumina, Inc, San Diego, CA, USA) or 454 Titanium (454 Life Sciences Corporation, Branford, CT, USA) for longer sequence reads

Fingerprinting: DGGE/TGGE: separates individual rRNA genes and provides a fingerprint of the complexity of the intestinal microbiota

T-RFLP: rapid comparative analysis and very sensitive

FISH: best for enumeration of species in the intestinal tract

PhyloChip (Affymetrix Corporation, Lawrence Berkeley Lab (LBNL), San Francisco, CA, USA): DNA microarray for multiple bacterial identification

for phylogenetic studies, because some regions of the gene encoding it are highly conserved and can act as primer binding sites, whereas other regions containing phylogenetic information are highly variable and enable their use for taxonomic classification. Using this approach, polymerase chain reaction (PCR) amplicons are sequenced using novel high-throughput pyrosequencing technology. Based on the degree of nucleotide similarity (usually between 95% and 99%), sequences can be binned into operational taxonomic units that form the basis for comparisons of microbiota composition and diversity between samples.

Although most of the initial efforts for taxonomic evaluation of the microbiome involved use of the 16S rRNA, more recent work has focused on sequencing of the genomes of the entire community using shotgun techniques that sequence the entire genome. Using this approach, Venter and colleagues[14] identified a vast number of microbes that had not previously been recognized to exist in the oceans. Over the past few years, similar techniques are being applied to the human intestinal microbiome, and with future refinement of the technology, bioinformatics, statistical analyses, and decreases in cost of the analyses should yield important new information about the microbes present in the intestine and how they relate to health and disease.

ADJUNCTS TO MICROBIOME ANALYSIS: FUNCTIONAL CHARACTERIZATION

Even if the taxonomy of a particular microbial community is identified, the functional expression as it relates to physiology and interaction with the host is not clarified. Simple identification of individual microbes or microbial genotypes often does not clarify their phenotypic expression. Thus, in addition to microbiome identification-based technologies, it is important to clarify the function of the microbial communities of interest within a particular niche. It thus is of interest to identify the mRNA and protein expression of the genes as well as the metabolites that result before and after interaction of the microbial gene products with the host. Additional "-omic" disciplines are thus being applied to augment studies of the microbiome (Box 2). Metatranscriptomics, metaproteinomics, and metabolomics identify gene expression products (mRNA), proteins, and metabolites resulting from the genes within a complex microbial community, such as that found in fecal sample.

Several metatranscriptome and metaproteome studies describing the human intestinal microbiota have confirmed the importance of bacterial functions related to carbohydrate metabolism in the colon. Similar results were seen in a transcriptional analysis of fecal samples from a monozygotic, obese twin pair[15] and metatranscriptomic

> **Box 2**
> **Studies of functional expression of the intestinal microbiome**
>
> Metagenomics (profiling intestinal microbiota, DNA): comparison with known functional expression of similar sequences
>
> Metabolomics: metabolic profiles (metabolites) associated with microbiota
>
> Metaproteomics: catalytic potential of microbiota (proteins)
>
> Metatranscriptomics: microbiota responses to environmental changes (RNA)

analysis of fecal samples from 10 healthy volunteers.[16] Metatranscriptomic data from the less studied small intestinal microbiota showed enrichment in sugar phosphotransferase (PTS) and other carbohydrate transport systems, as well as energy, central metabolic, and amino acid conversion pathways compared with the metagenome.[17] This finding suggests rapid uptake and fermentation of available simple sugars by the small intestinal microbiota, compared with the degradation of more complex carbohydrates by the bacteria in the colon. The importance of carbohydrate metabolism is also evident from the enormous amount of carbohydrate-active enzymes (CAZymes) present in the gut microbiome. Another recent study using fecal samples from studies of adult humans found that most assigned transcripts belonged to the metabolism cluster (26% of all sequences), underlining that even at the end of the intestinal tract the microbiota are still very active.[18]

Metaproteomics is the study of proteins collectively expressed within microbial communities that usually use mass spectrometry-based analyses to detect proteins associated with the microbiota identified within a given niche. These studies usually also use a systems-biology approach to evaluate the likely functions of the proteins produced by the microbiota. A recent study used a nontargeted, shotgun mass spectrometry-based whole-community proteomics, or metaproteomics, approach for the first deep proteome measurements of thousands of proteins in human fecal samples.[19] The resulting metaproteomes had a distribution that was unexpected relative to the metagenome, with more proteins for translation, energy production, and carbohydrate metabolism when compared with what was earlier predicted from metagenomics. Human proteins, including antimicrobial peptides, were also identified, providing a nontargeted glimpse of the host response to the microbiota. Several unknown proteins represented previously undescribed microbial pathways or host immune responses, revealing a novel complex interplay between the human host and its associated microbes.

The intestinal microbiota are involved in the regulation of multiple host metabolic pathways, giving rise to interactive host-microbiota metabolic, signaling, and immune-inflammatory processes connecting the intestine, liver, muscle, and brain.

These interactions begin at birth and likely even during fetal life. The microbiota shape the development of the immune system, and the immune system in turn shapes the composition of the microbiota through a cross-talk between the microbes and the host immune system. The signaling processes, together with direct chemical interactions between the microbe and host, act on multiple organs such as the gut, liver, muscle, and brain.

Fig. 2 summarizes some of the gut bacteria and the metabolites they contribute. Notable among these metabolites are the short-chain fatty acids (acetate, propionate, and butyrate), choline, bile acids, vitamin K, and polyamines, all believed to be important for optimal functioning of the gastrointestinal tract as well as the entire human. The production of these metabolites by microbes contributes to the host

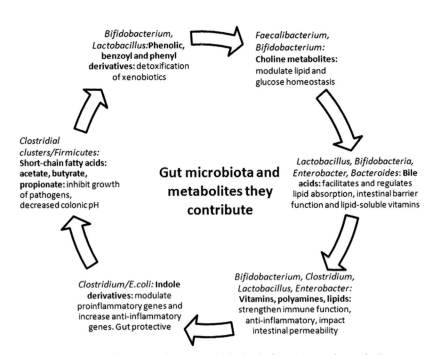

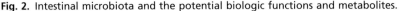

Fig. 2. Intestinal microbiota and the potential biologic functions and metabolites.

metabolic phenotype and hence to disease risk. Despite the putative importance of these metabolic functions, few studies are available as they pertain to NEC in the neonate.

ALTERATIONS OF THE INTESTINAL MICROBIOTA IN NEC

The intestinal microbiota normally exist in a commensal or symbiotic relationship with the host,[20] but in the neonate and especially in the premature infant, this relationship needs to develop, and many factors define its delicate equilibrium with the capability to modulate immune responses and promote health (**Fig. 3**).[21] As mentioned earlier, a specific pathogen that fulfills Koch's postulates for the cause of NEC has not been found. Whether the use of new-generation sequencing technologies will help in this search is unknown, although some preliminary studies are offering clues.

In a study by Wang and colleagues,[22] fecal samples from 20 preterm infants, 10 with NEC and 10 matched controls (including 4 twin pairs), were obtained from patients in a single-site level III neonatal intensive care unit. Bacterial DNA was subjected to terminal restriction fragment length polymorphism analysis and library sequencing of the 16S rRNA gene. The distribution of samples from patients with NEC distinctly clustered separately from controls. Intestinal bacterial colonization in all preterm infants was notable for low diversity. Patients with NEC had even less diversity, an increase in abundance of Gammaproteobacteria, a decrease in other bacteria species, and had received a higher mean number of previous days of antibiotics. These results suggested a relationship with previous use of antibiotics in patients with NEC. Whether the differences in clustering were because the samples were obtained at the time of NEC when these babies were receiving antibiotics is not clear.

In another study by Mai and colleagues,[23] starting with the first stool and continuing until discharge, weekly stool specimens were collected prospectively from infants

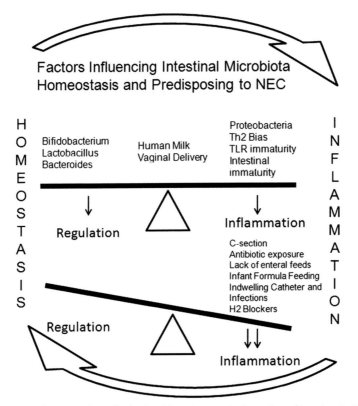

Fig. 3. Factors influencing intestinal microbiota homeostasis and predisposing to NEC. The intestinal microbiota are in perfect equilibrium with bacteria that regulate and others that have the potential to cause inflammation. Disruption of this equilibrium (dysbiosis) for different factors leads to inflammation.

with gestational ages 32 completed weeks or less or birth weights 1250 g or less. High-throughput 16S rRNA sequencing was used to compare the diversity of microbiota and the prevalence of specific bacterial signatures in 9 NEC infants and in 9 matched controls. A bloom (34% increase) of Proteobacteria and a decrease (32%) in Firmicutes in NEC cases between 1 week and less than 72 hours was detected. No significant change was identified in the controls. Several molecular signatures were identified to be increased in NEC cases 1 week before and within 72 hours of NEC development. One of the bacterial signatures detected more frequently in NEC cases ($P<.01$) matched closest to γ-Proteobacteria (similar to the Wang study[22]). Although this sequence grouped to the well-studied Enterobacteriaceae family, it did not match any sequence in GenBank by more than 97%. These observations suggest that abnormal patterns of microbiota and potentially a novel pathogen contribute to the cause of NEC.

FACTORS AFFECTING THE INTESTINAL MICROBIOTA
Prenatal

Thus, at this juncture, it seems that the microbiota of babies who subsequently develop NEC are different from those who do not. It will be important to dissect the factors that contribute to these differences, which may begin in fetal life (see **Fig. 3**). Recent PCR-based studies estimate the prevalence of microbial invasion of the amniotic cavity to be 30% to 50% higher than that detected by cultivation-based methods.[24] These studies have shown that cultivation-resistant anaerobes belonging to the family Fusobacteriaceae (particularly *Sneathia sanguinegens* and *Leptotrichia* spp) are also commonly found in amniotic fluid. Other diverse microbes detected by PCR of amniotic fluid include as-yet uncultivated and uncharacterized species. A causal relationship between diverse microbes, as detected by PCR, and preterm birth is supported by types of association (eg, space, time, and dose) proposed as alternatives to Koch's postulates for inferring causality from molecular findings. Whether this colonization affects the gastrointestinal tract of the fetus is not known, but the fact that the fetus swallows large quantities of amniotic fluid during the last trimester of pregnancy and the recent finding that microbial DNA is present in meconium suggest that the fetal intestine is exposed to the amniotic fluid microbes. The high sensitivity of the fetal intestine to inflammatory mediators such as lipopolysaccharide (LPS) suggests that in utero microbes may trigger intestinal inflammation in utero[25] Furthermore, it can be speculated that exposure of the intestinal tract to toll-like receptor (TLR) agonists such as LPS, flagellin, or microbial CpG in low quantities may also make the intestine tolerant to further inflammatory stimuli.[26]

Postnatal

Postnatally, many factors can influence intestinal bacterial colonization as well as the responses to colonization. Some studies have shown that mode of delivery (vaginal vs cesarean section), type of milk (human vs formula), and use of antibiotics influence the intestinal flora.[27–29] Those infants born via cesarean section, fed formula milk, and exposed to antibiotics have a decrease in diversity of intestinal microbiota and abnormal patterns of colonization, with suppression of healthy bacteria such as Lactobacillus and bifidobacteria.

Cesarean Section Versus Vaginal Delivery

Epidemiologic data showing a relationship between increased rate of cesarean section and risk for development of subsequent diseases was recently reviewed.[30] In the United States, the rate of cesarean delivery has increased 48% since 1996, reaching a level of 31.8% in 2007. This trend is reflected in many parts of the world, with the most populous country in the world, China, approaching 50% and some private clinics in Brazil approaching 80%. Concurrent with the trend of increasing deliveries by cesarean section, there has been an epidemic of both autoimmune diseases, such as type 1 diabetes, Crohn disease, and multiple sclerosis, and allergic diseases, such as asthma, allergic rhinitis, and atopic dermatitis. The occurrence of these diseases is higher in more affluent, Western, industrialized countries. As reviewed in Ref,[30] several previous studies have shown differences in microbial colonization after cesarean section and vaginal deliveries. A more recent study,[31] in which nonculture-based sequencing technology was used, examined the early stages of the colonization of the body by microbes. Babies born vaginally were colonized predominantly by *Lactobacillus*, whereas babies delivered by cesarean section were colonized by a mixture of potentially pathogenic bacteria typically found on the skin and in hospitals, such as *Staphylococcus* and *Acinetobacter*, suggesting that babies born by cesarean delivery were colonized with skin flora in lieu of the traditionally vaginal type of bacterium.[32] The data relating these changes to later outcomes such as celiac disease, allergies, and atopy are compelling, but a relationship of cesarean section versus vaginal delivery, intestinal colonization, and the development of NEC has not been found.

Human Milk Versus Infant Formula

Animal and human studies have shown that human milk decreases the incidence of NEC.[33–35] Beneficial factors of breast milk include immunoglobulins, cytokines, lactoferrin, lysozyme, and growth factors, but more importantly, healthy bacteria are promoted by human milk oligosaccharides (HMO).[27,36] HMOs contain a lactose core and act as prebiotics stimulating growth of *Bifidobacterium* species.[37,38] At birth, the rapid colonization of intestinal flora develops in the newborn first with aerobic or facultative anaerobic bacteria such as enterobacteria, enterococci, and staphylococci, and then during growth, they consume oxygen, allowing the proliferation of anaerobic bacteria such as *Bacteroides*, *Bifidobacterium*, and *Clostridium* species.[39,40] In the formula-fed infant, this transition tends to not occur that way and the newborn intestinal flora differs in its pattern of colonization with respect to breast-fed infants with predominance of gram-negatives and fewer anaerobes.[41,42] If they are grouped by phyla, breast-fed infants have predominance of Firmicutes mainly *Lactobacillus*, *Bacteroides* and Actinobacteria (*Bifidobacterium*) compared with formula-fed infants, who have predominance of Proteobacteria such as *Escherichia coli* and Firmicutes, some whom have pathogenic characteristics such as *Clostridium* and *Staphylococcus*. In 1 study, it was speculated that the abnormal pattern of colonization early at birth with delayed bloom of more pathogenic bacteria late in preterm infants could potentially explain those patients who develop NEC.[23] Sullivan and colleagues[33] in 1 multicenter study using donor human milk showed that an exclusively human milk-based diet is associated with significantly lower rates of NEC and surgical NEC when compared with a mother's milk-based diet that also includes bovine milk-based products. The reduction in NEC using strategies of only human milk was of 50% for clinical NEC and almost 90% for surgical NEC. The number needed to treat to prevent 1 case of NEC was estimated to be 10. In a recent policy statement by the American Academy of Pediatrics regarding breastfeeding and the use of human milk, the recommendation was to offer donor milk to all preterm infants in whom mother's own milk is unavailable.[43]

Antibiotic Exposure

The use of antibiotics is widespread in the neonatal intensive care unit (NICU). Often, their use is justified, but sometimes, it is the product of fear of infections in the preterm infant. Nevertheless, the use of antibiotics in neonates and especially in the preterm infant has unintended and sometimes devastating consequences. Antibiotic exposure may reduce the diversity of intestinal microbiota, delay the colonization of beneficial bacteria, and predispose preterm neonates to NEC. Previous studies[44–46] have shown that duration of antibiotic exposure is associated with an increased risk of NEC among neonates without previous sepsis. One study[47] found that overgrowth of pathogenic species is increased after 3 days of antimicrobial exposure. In the United States, most mothers giving birth prematurely are treated with antibiotics and many very-low-birth-weight infants are treated with a course of broad-spectrum antibiotics such as ampicillin and gentamicin. Studies[28] have shown the detrimental effects of antibiotics to the intestinal flora, even after 1 dose of antibiotics with alterations in the intestinal microbiota that could take years to recover. One study[48] showed a decrease in diversity, a predominance of less desirable bacteria and highly resistant clones with abundance of specific resistance genes as a result of antibiotic exposure that did not recover after 2 years after exposure. Cotten and colleagues[49] found that each empiric treatment day with antibiotic was associated with increased odds of death, NEC, and the composite measure of NEC or death. These investigators concluded that prolonged initial empiric antibiotic therapy may be associated with increased risk of NEC or death and should be used with caution.

Extreme caution should then be exerted at the moment of deciding to start antibiotics in preterm infants. Long-lasting consequences and life-threatening situations could result from the indiscriminate use of antibiotics.

INTESTINAL MICROBIOTA ALTERATION INDUCES INTESTINAL INFLAMMATION AND CYTOKINES

Immature intestinal response and alterations in the intestinal microbiota predispose the intestine of neonates to inflammation and to a cascade of proinflammatory and counterinflammatory cytokines response. Proinflammatory cytokines such as tumor necrosis factor (TNF), interleukin 1 (IL-1), IL-6, IL-8, endothelin 1, and platelet-activating factor are all increased in patients that develop NEC.[50–52]

The intestinal flora in the neonate have important functions in metabolism, nutrition, immune system, and defense against pathogens.[53,54] The immune system is developmentally regulated; therefore, in preterm babies, this immune system is still immature. Normally, it recognizes and fights harmful bacteria but does not react against healthy species of bacteria.[55,56] To avoid triggering pathologic immune responses, commensal bacteria must not express key virulence factors. For example, LPS is pentacylated in *Bacteroides* species, which are abundant in the intestinal flora of breast-fed, healthy infants. This modification makes lipid A in commensal *Bacteroides* a poor agonist of TLRs.[57] Conversely, lipid A of Proteobacteria is a potent agonist of TLR-4 and more likely to elicit an immune response because of its hexacylated characteristics.[58,59] The intestinal mucosa has mechanisms of recognition of bacterial products via highly specialized pattern recognition receptors called TLRs, which recognize specific microbial-associated molecular patterns (MAMPs).[60] Each MAMP has its own specific TLR.[61] For example, LPS, which acts as the endotoxin for gram-negative bacteria, is recognized by TLR-4. Flagellin is recognized by TLR-5, whereas peptidoglycan and lipotechoic acid from gram-positive bacteria are detected by TLR-2. TLR expression seems to be regulated by patterns of intestinal colonization, and therefore, abnormal patterns of colonization can trigger inappropriate responses. These MAMPs activate the specific TLR that leads to the activation of nuclear factor κ B (NF-κB) and caspases, which in turn activate transcription genes and induce cytokines such as IL-1, IL-6, IL-8, TNF-α, and interferon (IFN-1) (**Fig. 4**). Commensal healthy bacteria are believed to regulate this intestinal inflammatory response.[60,62] For example, studies have shown that *Lactobacillus* protects against cytokine-mediated cell injury.[63] *Bifidobacterium*, *Bacteroides thetaiotaomicron*, and *Streptococcus thermophilus* are examples of other bacteria that play a role in cytoprotection of the enterocyte and intestinal mucosa.[64] Many of these bacteria have been studied as therapeutic agents in the treatment of NEC, with promising results. Several studies, including a recent meta-analysis of the literature,[65,66] showed that the incidence of NEC was decreased in infants treated with probiotics containing different combination of these beneficial bacteria. Probiotics seems to help maintain a normal intestinal flora in neonates, thereby decreasing the incidence of NEC. Current evidence led to a recommendation level B in 2011 of effectiveness (recommendation is based on positive-controlled studies, but 1 negative study did not support the primary outcome).[67] Others[68,69] have suggested that dead microbes may be as effective as live microbes in modulating excessive inflammatory stimuli (see **Fig. 4**).

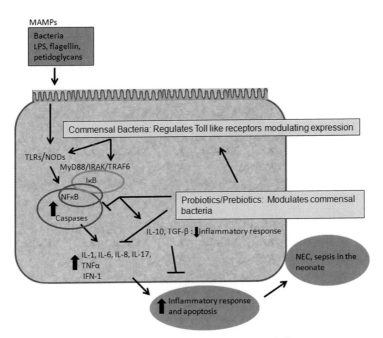

Fig. 4. Simplified TLR signaling leading to NF-κB activation, inflammatory response, and possible NEC. Surface enterocytes can recognize MAMPs via TLRs. Each of these receptors recognizes a specific bacterial product. For example, TLR-2 recognizes products of gram-positive bacteria, TLR-4 recognizes LPS from gram-negative bacteria, and TLR-5 recognizes flagellin. Cell stimulation signals recruitment of MyD88, IRAK, and TRAF6, then triggers activation of IκB. NF-κB activates the transcription of genes, including cytokines and chemokines. IκB: inhibitor of kappa B.

There are many opportunities for the physicians taking care of neonates to provide interventions that improve the adequate colonization of the neonatal gut and to minimize the deleterious but often unavoidable effects of medical treatment.

INTESTINAL MICROBIOTA BACTERIAL TRANSLOCATION AND OTHER RISK FACTORS FOR NEC

Bacterial translocation has been suggested as one of the mechanisms for developing NEC.[70,71] Bacterial translocation is not restricted only to the invasion of intestinal bacteria but can also include bacterial toxins or antigens that damage the intestinal epithelia and enter the circulation, resulting in a systemic inflammatory response.[72] During inflammation, production of nitric oxide alters expression and localization of the tight junction. Disruption of the tight junction zonulin proteins ZO-1, ZO-2, ZO-3, and occludin leads to intestinal permeability and bacterial translocation.[73] Few studies have shown the relationship between bacterial translocation and NEC. In 1 study[74] of bloodstream infections (BSIs) in very-low-birth-weight infants, BSI was more common after diagnosis of NEC in very-low-birth-weight infants who developed intestinal failure (60%) compared with those with surgical NEC without intestinal failure (42%) and those with medical NEC (20%). Coagulase-negative *Staphylococcus* and *Klebsiella* were the most frequently identified microorganisms. Alteration in the intestinal permeability was believed to be one of the mechanisms of BSI. Causation is difficult to establish. Nonculture-based analyses of intestinal microbiota have given us some indication of the alterations in diversity and intestinal flora composition of those infants who develop NEC.

However, what causes bacterial translocation? Bacterial translocation is believed to be secondary to abnormal intestinal colonization. Risk factors for bacterial translocation are discussed elsewhere in this article. Other factors have been associated with increased risk of NEC probably secondary to bacterial trans-location. Histamine 2 (H_2) blockers, which are sometimes used in NICUs, have been shown to increase the risk of sepsis and meningitis.[75] It seems that increasing the gastric pH in preterm infants predisposes the neonate to bacterial translocation and infection.[76] Guillet and colleagues[75] showed in their study that those infants less than 1500 g treated with H_2 blocker were more likely to develop NEC. In a study performed several years ago, Carrion and Egan[77] reported that by main-taining an acidic gastric pH less than 3.0, the incidence of NEC decreased and higher gastric enteric bacterial colony counts were strongly correlated with gastric pH level of more than 4.

REFERENCES

1. Obladen M. Necrotizing enterocolitis–150 years of fruitless search for the cause. Neonatology 2009;96(4):203–10.
2. Neu J, Walker WA. Necrotizing enterocolitis. N Engl J Med 2011;364(3):255–64.
3. Lin Patricia W, Stoll Barbara J. Necrotising enterocolitis. Lancet 2006;368(9543): 1271–83.
4. Young CM, Kingma SD, Neu J. Ischemia-reperfusion and neonatal intestinal injury. J Pediatr 2011;158(2 Suppl):e25–8.
5. Claud EC, Walker WA. Hypothesis: inappropriate colonization of the premature intestine can cause neonatal necrotizing enterocolitis. FASEB J 2001;15(8): 1398–403.
6. Sántulli TV, Schullinger JN, Heird WC, et al. Acute necrotizing enterocolitis in infancy: a review of 64 cases. Pediatrics 1975;55(3):376–87.
7. Falkow S. Molecular Koch's postulates applied to bacterial pathogenicity–a personal recollection 15 years later. Nat Rev Microbiol 2004;2(1):67–72.
8. Resta S, Luby JP, Rosenfeld CR, et al. Isolation and propagation of a human enteric coronavirus. Science 1985;229(4717):978–81.
9. Neu J, Mshvildadze M, Mai V. A roadmap for understanding and preventing necrotizing enterocolitis. Curr Gastroenterol Rep 2008;10(5):450–7.
10. Grave GD, Nelson SA, Walker WA, et al. New therapies and preventive approaches for necrotizing enterocolitis: report of a research planning workshop. Pediatr Res 2007;62(4):510–4.
11. Ben-Amor K, Heilig H, Smidt H, et al. Genetic diversity of viable, injured, and dead fecal bacteria assessed by fluorescence-activated cell sorting and 16S rRNA gene analysis. Appl Environ Microbiol 2005;71(8):4679–89.
12. Leblond-Bourget N, Philippe H, Mangin I, et al. 16S rRNA and 16S to 23S internal transcribed spacer sequence analyses reveal inter- and intraspecific Bifidobacterium phylogeny. Int J Syst Bacteriol 1996;46(1):102–11.
13. Rondon MR, August PR, Bettermann AD, et al. Cloning the soil metagenome: a strategy for accessing the genetic and functional diversity of uncultured micro-organisms. Appl Environ Microbiol 2000;66(6):2541–7.
14. Venter JC, Remington K, Heidelberg JF, et al. Environmental genome shotgun sequencing of the Sargasso Sea. Science 2004;304(5667):66–74.

15. Turnbaugh PJ, Quince C, Faith JJ, et al. Organismal, genetic, and transcriptional variation in the deeply sequenced gut microbiomes of identical twins. Proc Natl Acad Sci U S A 2010;107(16):7503–8.
16. Gosalbes MJ, Durban A, Pignatelli M, et al. Metatranscriptomic approach to analyze the functional human gut microbiota. PLoS One 2011;6(3):e17447.
17. Zoetendal EG, Raes J, van den Bogert B, et al. The human small intestinal microbiota is driven by rapid uptake and conversion of simple carbohydrates. ISME J 2012;6(7):1415–26.
18. Booijink CC, Boekhorst J, Zoetendal EG, et al. Metatranscriptome analysis of the human fecal microbiota reveals subject-specific expression profiles, with genes encoding proteins involved in carbohydrate metabolism being dominantly expressed. Appl Environ Microbiol 2010;76(16):5533–40.
19. Verberkmoes NC, Russell AL, Shah M, et al. Shotgun metaproteomics of the human distal gut microbiota. ISME J 2009;3(2):179–89.
20. Hooper LV, Gordon JI. Commensal host-bacterial relationships in the gut. Science 2001;292(5519):1115–8.
21. Forsythe P, Bienenstock J. Immunomodulation by commensal and probiotic bacteria. Immunol Invest 2010;39(4–5):429–48.
22. Wang Y, Hoenig JD, Malin KJ, et al. 16S rRNA gene-based analysis of fecal microbiota from preterm infants with and without necrotizing enterocolitis. ISME J 2009;3(8):944–54.
23. Mai V, Young CM, Ukhanova M, et al. Fecal microbiota in premature infants prior to necrotizing enterocolitis. PLoS One 2011;6(6):e20647.
24. DiGiulio DB, Gervasi MT, Romero R, et al. Microbial invasion of the amniotic cavity in pregnancies with small-for-gestational-age fetuses. J Perinat Med 2010;38(5):495–502.
25. Nanthakumar NN, Fusunyan RD, Sanderson I, et al. Inflammation in the developing human intestine: a possible pathophysiologic contribution to necrotizing enterocolitis. Proc Natl Acad Sci U S A 2000;97(11):6043–8.
26. Medzhitov R, Schneider DS, Soares MP. Disease tolerance as a defense strategy. Science 2012;335(6071):936–41.
27. Harmsen HJ, Wildeboer-Veloo AC, Raangs GC, et al. Analysis of intestinal flora development in breast-fed and formula-fed infants by using molecular identification and detection methods. J Pediatr Gastroenterol Nutr 2000;30(1):61–7.
28. Jernberg C, Lofmark S, Edlund C, et al. Long-term ecological impacts of antibiotic administration on the human intestinal microbiota. ISME J 2007;1(1):56–66.
29. Gronlund MM, Lehtonen OP, Eerola E, et al. Fecal microflora in healthy infants born by different methods of delivery: permanent changes in intestinal flora after cesarean delivery. J Pediatr Gastroenterol Nutr 1999;28(1):19–25.
30. Neu J, Rushing J. Cesarean versus vaginal delivery: long-term infant outcomes and the hygiene hypothesis. Clin Perinatol 2011;38(2):321–31.
31. Dominguez-Bello MG, Blaser MJ, Ley RE, et al. Development of the human gastrointestinal microbiota and insights from high-throughput sequencing. Gastroenterology 2011;140(6):1713–9.
32. Dominguez-Bello MG, Costello EK, Contreras M, et al. Delivery mode shapes the acquisition and structure of the initial microbiota across multiple body habitats in newborns. Proc Natl Acad Sci U S A 2010;107(26):11971–5.
33. Sullivan S, Schanler RJ, Kim JH, et al. An exclusively human milk-based diet is associated with a lower rate of necrotizing enterocolitis than a diet of human milk and bovine milk-based products. J Pediatr 2010;156(4):562–567.e1.
34. Barlow B, Santulli TV, Heird WC, et al. An experimental study of acute neonatal enterocolitis–the importance of breast milk. J Pediatr Surg 1974;9(5):587–95.

35. Lucas A, Cole TJ. Breast milk and neonatal necrotising enterocolitis. Lancet 1990; 336(8730):1519–23.
36. Hanson LA, Korotkova M, Telemo E. Breast-feeding, infant formulas, and the immune system. Ann Allergy Asthma Immunol 2003;90(6 Suppl 3):59–63.
37. Ward RE, Ninonuevo M, Mills DA, et al. In vitro fermentation of breast milk oligo-saccharides by *Bifidobacterium infantis* and *Lactobacillus gasseri*. Appl Environ Microbiol 2006;72(6):4497–9.
38. Ninonuevo MR, Park Y, Yin H, et al. A strategy for annotating the human milk glycome. J Agric Food Chem 2006;54(20):7471–80.
39. Adlerberth I, Lindberg E, Aberg N, et al. Reduced enterobacterial and increased staphylococcal colonization of the infantile bowel: an effect of hygienic lifestyle? Pediatr Res 2006;59(1):96–101.
40. Bjorkstrom MV, Hall L, Soderlund S, et al. Intestinal flora in very low-birth weight infants. Acta Paediatr 2009;98(11):1762–7.
41. Le Huerou-Luron I, Blat S, Boudry G. Breast- v. formula-feeding: impacts on the digestive tract and immediate and long-term health effects. Nutr Res Rev 2010; 23(1):23–36.
42. Penders J, Thijs C, Vink C, et al. Factors influencing the composition of the intestinal microbiota in early infancy. Pediatrics 2006;118(2):511–21.
43. Section on Breastfeeding. Breastfeeding and the use of human milk. Pediatrics 2012;129(3):e827–41.
44. Kuppala VS, Meinzen-Derr J, Morrow AL, et al. Prolonged initial empirical antibiotic treatment is associated with adverse outcomes in premature infants. J Pediatr 2011;159(5):720–5.
45. Alexander VN, Northrup V, Bizzarro MJ. Antibiotic exposure in the newborn intensive care unit and the risk of necrotizing enterocolitis. J Pediatr 2011;159(3): 392–7.
46. Weintraub AS, Ferrara L, Deluca L, et al. Antenatal antibiotic exposure in preterm infants with necrotizing enterocolitis. J Perinatol 2012;32(9):705–9.
47. Goldmann DA, Leclair J, Macone A. Bacterial colonization of neonates admitted to an intensive care environment. J Pediatr 1978;93(2):288–93.
48. Jakobsson HE, Jernberg C, Andersson AF, et al. Short-term antibiotic treatment has differing long-term impacts on the human throat and gut microbiome. PLoS One 2010;5(3):e9836.
49. Cotten CM, Taylor S, Stoll B, et al. Prolonged duration of initial empirical antibiotic treatment is associated with increased rates of necrotizing enterocolitis and death for extremely low birth weight infants. Pediatrics 2009;123(1):58–66.
50. Caplan MS, MacKendrick W. Necrotizing enterocolitis: a review of pathogenetic mechanisms and implications for prevention. Pediatr Pathol 1993;13(3): 357–69.
51. Caplan MS, Sun XM, Hseuh W, et al. Role of platelet activating factor and tumor necrosis factor-alpha in neonatal necrotizing enterocolitis. J Pediatr 1990;116(6): 960–4.
52. Edelson MB, Bagwell CE, Rozycki HJ. Circulating pro- and counterinflammatory cytokine levels and severity in necrotizing enterocolitis. Pediatrics 1999;103(4 Pt 1): 766–71.
53. Round JL, Mazmanian SK. The gut microbiota shapes intestinal immune responses during health and disease. Nat Rev Immunol 2009;9(5):313–23.
54. Murgas Torrazza R, Neu J. The developing intestinal microbiome and its relationship to health and disease in the neonate. J Perinatol 2011;31(Suppl 1):S29–34.

55. Rook GA. 99th Dahlem conference on infection, inflammation and chronic inflammatory disorders: Darwinian medicine and the 'hygiene' or 'old friends' hypothesis. Clin Exp Immunol 2010;160(1):70–9.
56. Macpherson AJ, Harris NL. Interactions between commensal intestinal bacteria and the immune system. Nat Rev Immunol 2004;4(6):478–85.
57. Coats SR, Do CT, Karimi-Naser LM, et al. Antagonistic lipopolysaccharides block E. coli lipopolysaccharide function at human TLR4 via interaction with the human MD-2 lipopolysaccharide binding site. Cell Microbiol 2007;9(5):1191–202.
58. Sansonetti PJ, Medzhitov R. Learning tolerance while fighting ignorance. Cell 2009;138(3):416–20.
59. Munford RS, Varley AW. Shield as signal: lipopolysaccharides and the evolution of immunity to gram-negative bacteria. PLoS Pathog 2006;2(6):e67.
60. Sharma R, Young C, Neu J. Molecular modulation of intestinal epithelial barrier: contribution of microbiota. J Biomed Biotechnol 2010;2010:305879.
61. Rhee SH. Basic and translational understandings of microbial recognition by toll-like receptors in the intestine. J Neurogastroenterol Motil 2011;17(1):28–34.
62. Caplan MS. Probiotic and prebiotic supplementation for the prevention of neonatal necrotizing enterocolitis. J Perinatol 2009;29(Suppl 2):S2–6.
63. Tien MT, Girardin SE, Regnault B, et al. Anti-inflammatory effect of Lactobacillus casei on Shigella-infected human intestinal epithelial cells. J Immunol 2006; 176(2):1228–37.
64. Otte JM, Podolsky DK. Functional modulation of enterocytes by gram-positive and gram-negative microorganisms. Am J Physiol Gastrointest Liver Physiol 2004;286(4):G613–26.
65. Lin HC, Hsu CH, Chen HL, et al. Oral probiotics prevent necrotizing enterocolitis in very low birth weight preterm infants: a multicenter, randomized, controlled trial. Pediatrics 2008;122(4):693–700.
66. Deshpande G, Rao S, Patole S, et al. Updated meta-analysis of probiotics for preventing necrotizing enterocolitis in preterm neonates. Pediatrics 2010;125(5): 921–30.
67. Floch MH, Walker WA, Madsen K, et al. Recommendations for probiotic use-2011 update. J Clin Gastroenterol 2011;45(Suppl):S168–71.
68. Zhang L, Li N, Caicedo R, et al. Alive and dead Lactobacillus rhamnosus GG decrease tumor necrosis factor-alpha-induced interleukin-8 production in Caco-2 cells. J Nutr 2005;135(7):1752–6.
69. Zhang L, Li N, des Robert C, et al. Lactobacillus rhamnosus GG decreases lipopolysaccharide-induced systemic inflammation in a gastrostomy-fed infant rat model. J Pediatr Gastroenterol Nutr 2006;42(5):545–52.
70. Sherman MP. New concepts of microbial translocation in the neonatal intestine: mechanisms and prevention. Clin Perinatol 2010;37(3):565–79.
71. Hunter CJ, Upperman JS, Ford HR, et al. Understanding the susceptibility of the premature infant to necrotizing enterocolitis (NEC). Pediatr Res 2008;63(2): 117–23.
72. Gatt M, Reddy BS, MacFie J. Review article: bacterial translocation in the critically ill-evidence and methods of prevention. Aliment Pharmacol Ther 2007; 25(7):741–57.
73. Anand RJ, Leaphart CL, Mollen KP, et al. The role of the intestinal barrier in the pathogenesis of necrotizing enterocolitis. Shock 2007;27(2):124–33.
74. Cole CR, Hansen NI, Higgins RD, et al. Bloodstream infections in very low birth weight infants with intestinal failure. J Pediatr 2012;160(1):54–59.e2.

75. Guillet R, Stoll BJ, Cotten CM, et al. Association of H2-blocker therapy and higher incidence of necrotizing enterocolitis in very low birth weight infants. Pediatrics 2006;117(2):e137–42.
76. Canani RB, Terrin G. Gastric acidity inhibitors and the risk of intestinal infections. Curr Opin Gastroenterol 2010;26(1):31–5.
77. Carrion V, Egan EA. Prevention of neonatal necrotizing enterocolitis. J Pediatr Gastroenterol Nutr 1990;11(3):317–23.

Inflammatory Signaling in Necrotizing Enterocolitis

Isabelle G. De Plaen, MD

KEYWORDS

- Necrotizing enterocolitis • Inflammatory mediators • Inflammation • TLR • Cytokines
- Chemokines • PAF • NO - ROS

KEY POINTS

- The pathogenesis of necrotizing enterocolitis (NEC) remains poorly defined and is likely attributable to a complex mechanism.
- The production of many inflammatory mediators is developmentally regulated in the intestine.
- Immaturities of several pathways that regulate inflammation may predispose premature infants to inflammation.
- Excessive inflammation may play an important role in NEC.

INTRODUCTION

The pathogenesis of necrotizing enterocolitis (NEC) remains poorly understood. Many factors potentially predispose the premature intestine to injury: (1) a lack of adequate substrate and O2 delivery to the intestinal epithelial cells because of an incomplete microvasculature development or to an immature regulation of the intestinal vascular tone; (2) an inadequate intestinal barrier; (3) an inflammatory response triggered by abnormal bacterial colonization; and (4) an immature immune response leading to inefficient killing of microbes that then translocate through the epithelium (**Fig. 1**). At the same time, an excessive production of inflammatory mediators leads to the recruitment of neutrophils and subsequent tissue injury and necrosis.

The pathogenesis of NEC is complex and its speed of progression is quite variable. In an attempt to gain understanding of the disease, researchers have examined tissues resected from patients with NEC; however, as these are obtained at late stages of the disease, they do not yield clues about the early pathogenic events leading to NEC. Therefore, animal models have been used and have helped to identify a role

Division of Neonatology, Department of Pediatrics, Children's Hospital of Chicago Research Center, Ann and Robert H. Lurie Children's Hospital of Chicago, Northwestern University Feinberg School of Medicine, 225 East Chicago Avenue, Box 45, Chicago, IL 60611-2605, USA
E-mail address: isabelledp@northwestern.edu

Clin Perinatol 40 (2013) 109–124
http://dx.doi.org/10.1016/j.clp.2012.12.008
0095-5108/13/$ – see front matter © 2013 Elsevier Inc. All rights reserved.
perinatology.theclinics.com

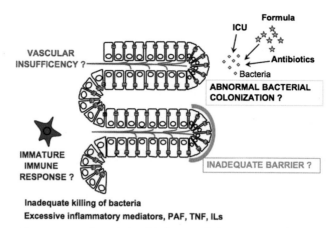

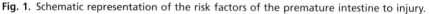

Fig. 1. Schematic representation of the risk factors of the premature intestine to injury.

for several mediators of the inflammatory network in NEC. In this article, we discuss the evidence for the role of these inflammatory mediators and conclude with a current unifying hypothesis regarding NEC pathogenesis.

BACTERIAL–LIPOPOLYSACCHARIDE

During the birth process, the newborn intestine is exposed to the many microbes from the environment and colonization occurs. In term infants, the intestine is colonized with microbes derived from the maternal birth canal and the environment. Exposure to breast milk induces the development of a rich balanced microflora and the growth of *bifidobacteria*, which have many protective properties for the neonatal gut. Compared with full-term infants, the colonization process in preterm infants is altered, as the growth of fewer but more aggressive bacteria[1] is facilitated by the lack of breast milk, the use of antibiotics and anti-acid medications,[2] and the neonatal intensive care unit (NICU) environment. This flora contains more "proinflammatory" bacteria and fewer commensals, which are known to induce genes that promote the epithelial barrier, digesting enzymes, and angiogenesis.[3] Bacterial overgrowth is further facilitated by the immaturities of intestinal motility and digestion, the intestinal barrier, and innate immunity. There is evidence that bacteria play a role in acute bowel injury in animal models. For example, germ-free rats were protected against injury in a model of acute bowel injury induced by platelet-activating factor (PAF).[4] In humans, an abnormal intestinal microflora skewed toward gram-negative bacteria has been found to be associated with the early stage of NEC.[5] Gram-negative bacteria contain lipopolysaccharides (LPS or endotoxin) on their outer membranes. LPS is a potent activator of the host immune response and may play a central role in NEC. LPS, when injected to rats and mice, produces intestinal injury and shock.[6] Increased serum LPS has been found in patients with NEC.[7] LPS is a potent activator of the transcription factor nuclear factor-κB (NF-κB)[8] and stimulates the production of many cytokines, including interleukin (IL)-1, IL-6, chemokines, tumor necrosis factor (TNF),[9] and PAF,[10] which all amplify the inflammatory response.

CYTOKINES: INFLAMMATION

The intestinal epithelial cells (IECs) are in contact with bacteria and their products. The bacterial-IEC interaction may be facilitated in the premature intestine by bacterial overgrowth and by an immature mucous layer. Components of the bacteria (called microbial-associated molecular patterns [MAMPs]) interact with Toll-like receptors (TLRs) on the IEC and on the submucosal inflammatory cells. Once activated, TLRs elicit the activation of several signal transduction pathways, including the inhibitor of NF-κB (IκB) kinase (IKK),[11] a critical upstream kinase that activates NF-κB, a major regulator of inflammation. This leads to the production of many inflammatory mediators, including cytokines and chemokines, which lead to immune cell recruitment, especially neutrophils, and to intestinal inflammation.

There are several pieces of evidence that suggest a role for excessive inflammation in NEC: (1) in patients with the disease, several cytokines have been found to be increased in the plasma and intestinal tissue[12,13]; (2) the incidence of NEC is decreased by prenatal use of glucocorticoids,[14] which are known potent inhibitors of the inflammatory response; (3) the production of IL-8 by enterocytes is developmentally regulated[15]; and (4) blocking the activation of NF-κB in a neonatal rat model protects against NEC.[16]

NF-κB

NF-κB is a transcription factor that regulates the expression of many proinflammatory cytokines, chemokines, and leukocyte adhesion molecules.[17,18] It consists of 5 subunits (p50, p65, p52, cRel, and RelB) that homo- or heterodimerize to form active NF-κB.[17,18] The dimers of NF-κB mostly found in intestinal tissues are p50-p50 and p50-p65.[19,20] NF-κB is constitutively present in the cytoplasm of most cells, bound to inhibitory proteins IκBs (**Fig. 2**). Following stimulation, IκB is phosphorylated by the upstream IKK complex.[17] This complex consists of 2 catalytic subunits, IKKα and IKKβ, and a regulatory component, NEMO (NF-κB essential modulator).[21] Phosphorylation of IκB by the IKK complex leads to its ubiquitination and subsequent degradation by the 26S proteasome, leaving NF-κB free to translocate to the nucleus and regulate the gene expression of many inflammatory mediators.[17,21] Our laboratory has shown that NF-κB is constitutively present at low levels in adult rat intestine, and is activated in PAF-induced acute bowel injury.[19] We also found that, in fetal rat intestines, the constitutive NF-κB activation appears at 20 days of gestation (length of gestation: 21 days).[16]

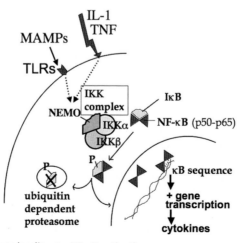

Fig. 2. Signaling events leading to NF-κB activation.

NF-κB has multiple functions in the intestine, some protective, others potentially detrimental. Several interventions known to decrease NEC, such as breastfeeding and use of probiotics, attenuate IEC NF-κB activation[22,23]: breast milk induces the production of IκBα in IECs[22] and probiotics inhibit NF-κB activation through the proteasome.[23] Mice with deletion of IKKβ in IECs are protected against systemic inflammation and multiple organ dysfunction syndromes following intestinal ischemia-reperfusion[24]; however, in several in vivo models, the activation of IKKβ and NF-κB in IECs has been shown to be protective and to limit intestinal mucosal damage.[24–26] Therefore, NF-κB in IECs might have both protective and detrimental properties in the intestine.

Previous work done in animal models by our laboratory and others suggests a role for NF-κB in NEC. In a neonatal rat NEC model, increased NEC severity (by histology) correlated with increased IEC staining for TLR-2 and activated NF-κB, as well as increased IEC apoptosis and impaired IEC proliferation.[27] We have shown that NF-κB is persistently activated in the intestine in a neonatal rat model of NEC[16] and neonatal rats treated with a specific NF-κB inhibitory peptide, but not a control peptide, had decreased mortality and bowel injury,[16] suggesting a central role for NF-κB in NEC. This same NF-κB inhibitory peptide inhibits LPS-induced chemokine CXCL2 (or MIP-2) gene expression in IECs[28] and inhibits LPS-induced interleukin-1β (IL-1β), IL-6, and TNF-alpha gene expression in the J774.1 murine macrophage-like cell line in vitro.[29]

There is evidence that NF-κB is developmentally regulated with higher activation and cytokine production in immature IECs[15] and inflammatory cells.[30,31] Intestinal NF-κB is strongly activated at birth, and is downregulated within a day in dam-fed newborn rats.[16] In contrast, NF-κB remains strongly activated at both day 1 (D1) and D2 in stressed animals and this is accompanied by a significant decrease in the levels of the endogenous NF-κB inhibitory proteins IκBα and IκBβ at D2.[16] Immature enterocytes expressed lower levels of specific IkappaB genes compared with mature enterocytes[15] and had a higher IL-8 response to bacterial infection.[15]

Although activation of NF-κB is an essential component of host immunity against pathogens,[32] in premature infants, a marked and prolonged NF-κB activation may contribute to intestinal tissue injury.[16]

TLR

TLRs are receptors for bacterial products (also called microbial-associated molecular patterns [MAMPs]), and are found on many cells, including IECs and inflammatory cells. Ten different TLRs have been identified to date in humans. In the intestine, when MAMPs, generally from commensal bacteria, interact with TLRs located on the intestinal epithelium, epithelial cell proliferation, immunoglobulin A (IgA) production, integrity of tight junctions, and antimicrobial peptide production are promoted, all of which help in maintaining a healthy intestinal barrier.[33] The interaction of MAMPs with TLRs on underlying lamina propria immune cells[33] can trigger a proinflammatory response, however. The location of these interactions may influence the response: apical exposure of IECs with CpG-DNA results in inhibition of NF-κB activation, whereas basolateral exposure leads to activation of NF-κB.[34] This suggests that invasive bacteria that can penetrate the epithelial barrier elicit a proinflammatory response at the basolateral site, whereas bacteria that cannot cross the barrier, generally nonpathogenic bacteria, remaining on the apical site, elicit a homeostatic, anti-inflammatory response.[33]

Murine and human NEC has been associated with increased intestinal TLR2 and TLR4[35] and decreased TLR9 expression.[36]

TLR4 is the receptor for endotoxin. Although a study found that TLR4 was protective in ischemia/reperfusion injury in neonatal mice,[37] there are many pieces of evidence that suggest that TLR4 has an injurious role in NEC: (1) intestinal TLR4 gene expression is increased in animals exposed to formula feeding and cold asphyxia stress during experimental NEC, whereas it is normally downregulated in dam-fed animals during the first 72 hours of life[38]; and (2) TLR4-deficient mice are protected against NEC.[38,39] TLR4 activation in IECs has been found to delay mucosal repair by inducing HMGB1 signaling, which increases stress fibers and focal adhesions[40] and reduces enterocyte proliferation by inhibiting beta-catenin signaling.[41]

Although the activation of TLR4 contributes to NEC, TLR9, a cell receptor for unmethylated CpG dinucleotides originated from bacterial DNA, has been shown to be protective. Indeed, TLR9-deficient mice exhibited increased NEC severity[36] and the activation of TLR9 by its ligand CpG-DNA inhibits LPS-mediated TLR4 signaling in enterocytes and reduces NEC severity.[36]

Interferon Gamma

Interferon gamma (or type II interferon) (IFNγ) is a cytokine produced mainly by T cells and natural killer cells, but also by B cells, NK-T cells, dendritic cells, and macrophages.[42] IFNγ is produced by macrophages early during infection. Its synthesis is induced in response to IL-12 and IL-18 and is inhibited by IL-4, IL-10, TGFβ, and glucocorticoids.[42] IFNγ activates several signaling pathways, including STAT1, PI-3kinase/Akt, and MAPKs, which regulate the transcription of more than 500 genes in the cell that modulate several cellular functions, such as apoptosis, proliferation, leukocyte migration, and epithelial permeability.[42]

A role for IFNγ in NEC has been suggested by the following evidence: a trend toward an increase in IFNγ in ileal tissues has been shown in experimental NEC.[43] IFNγ knock-out mice are protected against NEC and show increased epithelial cell restitution compared with wild-type controls when exposed to the NEC model.[44] IFNγ has been shown to inhibit enterocyte migration by reversibly displacing connexin43 from lipid rafts.[45]

IL-6

IL-6 is a cytokine produced by macrophages, T cells, and endothelial cells under the control of NF-κB. IL-6 triggers the production of acute-phase proteins in the liver, B-cell proliferation, and antibody production. IL-6 levels have been found to be elevated in the plasma and the stools of patients with NEC[46] and correlated with the severity of disease.[12]

IL-8

IL-8 is a chemokine produced by macrophages, endothelial cells, and epithelial cells. IL-8 is a potent chemoattractant for neutrophils and an angiogenic factor. IL-8 has been shown to be elevated in the plasma of infants with NEC[47] and to correlate with disease severity.[47] Fetal enterocytes have upregulated IL-8 gene expression compared with mature enterocytes,[15] which might contribute to the susceptibility of the premature intestine to inflammation.

IL-10

IL-10 is a cytokine secreted by Th2-cells that inhibits cytokine production in macrophages and other antigen presenting cells (APCs).[48] IL-10 modulates both innate and adaptive immune responses[48] and is a major anti-inflammatory cytokine in the intestine. In humans, IL-10 has been found to be increased in infants with severe

NEC,[47] which could be a compensatory mechanism to attenuate the intestinal inflammatory response. A role for IL-10 in NEC is suggested by the following work: IL-10–deficient mice are predisposed to inflammatory colitis.[49] The production of IL-10 by stimulated blood mononuclear leukocytes is diminished in the premature infant compared with the term infant[50] and may increase the susceptibility of the premature infant to inflammation. IL-10 levels were more frequently not detectable in the breast milk of premature infants who developed NEC compared with those who did not.[51] In a mouse model of NEC, IL-10 has been shown to be protective against NEC by attenuating the degree of intestinal inflammation, epithelial apoptosis, decreased junctional adhesion molecule-1 localization, and increased intestinal inducible nitric oxide synthase expression.[52]

IL-12

IL-12 is a cytokine released by macrophages, neutrophils, B cells, and dendritic cells in response to bacteria, viruses, and their products. It induces IFNγ and activates Th1 cells and macrophages. Although one study found that IL-12 is downregulated in NEC,[43] another has shown that IL-12 is upregulated in the ileum of neonatal rats with NEC, which correlates with the progression of the tissue damage.[53]

IL-18

IL-18, a proinflammatory cytokine released by macrophages, dendritic cells, and IECs, induces the production of IL-1β, IL-8, TNF-alpha, and IFNγ by inflammatory cells. Several pieces of evidence suggest an involvement of IL-18 in NEC: (1) a polymorphism of IL-18 has been associated with NEC[54]; (2) IL-18 is upregulated in the ileum of neonatal rats with NEC[53,55]; and (3) IL-18 knock-out mice have been shown to have decreased incidence of NEC.[56] They were also found to have higher levels of IkappaB-alpha and IkappaB-beta, suggesting less NF-κB activation.[56] They were also shown to have fewer ileal macrophages.[56]

TNF-alpha

TNF-alpha has been shown to mediate inflammatory bowel disease in adults.[57] Although TNF-alpha levels have not been found to be consistently increased in the plasma of infants with NEC,[12,46,58] TNF-alpha protein has been found to be increased in resected NEC intestinal tissues.[59] When examined by in situ hybridization, tissue obtained from patients with NEC had a marked increase in TNF-alpha mRNA in Paneth cells, as well as in infiltrating eosinophils and macrophages.[60] TNF-alpha has been found to be increased in a model of bowel injury in neonatal rats induced by hypoxia/reoxygenation[61] but not in a neonatal rat NEC model.[43] Our laboratory also did not find any increase in intestinal TNF-alpha in the neonatal rat NEC model (Liu SXL, 2008, unpublished data). Two independent studies found that anti–TNF-alpha antibodies improved the intestinal injury in a neonatal rat NEC model.[62,63] Also, pentoxifylline, a drug with many effects, including TNF-alpha inhibition, has been shown to decrease the incidence of NEC in neonatal rats.[64] However, our laboratory did not find any protective effect of anti-TNF in both a model of acute bowel injury induced by PAF and in a neonatal rat NEC model in which we compared rats treated with anti-TNF antibodies versus control immunoglobulin (Liu SXL, 2008, unpublished data). TNF-alpha has been shown to cause a marked loss of mucous-containing goblet cells in immature mice.[65] TNF-alpha causes apoptosis in IECs via production of mitochondrial ROS (reactive oxygen species) and activation of the JNK/p38 signaling pathway.[59]

PAF

PAF is an endogenous phospholipid mediator released by many cells, including neutrophils, mast cells, eosinophils, macrophages, platelets, endothelial cells, and bacteria, including *Escherichia coli*.[66–68] PAF binds to a G protein–coupled receptor, PAF-R, preferentially expressed in the ileum, but also abundant in the jejunum and the spleen.[69] PAF-R is present in many cells (eg, neutrophils, macrophages, and epithelial cells).[69,70] Activation of PAF-R causes a prolonged effect in vivo by the activation of a downstream cascade (eg, activation of NF-κB[19] and of PI3kinase/Akt[71]), and the production of endogenous PAF (by phospholipase A2 [PLA2]),[72] oxygen radicals by xanthine oxidase (a major oxidant producing enzyme in the small intestine),[73] and TNF-alpha.[74] In vivo, free PAF is rapidly degraded by its degrading enzyme, PAF-acetylhydrolase (PAF-AH). PAF has been shown to play an important role in NEC: (1) PAF-receptor antagonists prevent experimental NEC in a neonatal rat model[75] and in a piglet model,[76] and PAF-AH prevents experimental NEC in rats[77]; (2) infants with NEC have elevated circulating PAF[78] and decreased amounts of plasma PAF-AH,[79] compared with age-matched controls; (3) PAF-AH is present in human milk[80]; (4) intravenous infusion of recombinant PAF-AH prevents NEC in rats,[81] and PAF-AH knock-out mice are more susceptible to NEC, although their survival is higher[82]; and (5) the ileum, the site of predilection of NEC, has the highest amounts of PAF-R.[69] PAF also mediates the intestinal injury induced by hypoxia/reperfusion,[83] TNF-alpha,[84] and LPS.[85] Exogenous administration of PAF induces systemic hypotension, increased vascular permeability, hemoconcentration, and a dose-dependent isolated bowel necrosis,[86] which predominates in the small intestine (frequently the ileum) as seen in NEC. Therefore, PAF administration has been used as a model of acute bowel necrosis and NEC.[86] LPS administration potentiates PAF-induced bowel injury[6] and PAF mediates LPS[87] and hypoxia-induced bowel necrosis.[87] When injected intravenously, even at a dose below that which causes bowel necrosis, PAF activates NF-κB very rapidly (within 5 minutes, peaking at 30 minutes)[19] and induces the release of leukotrienes C4,[88] the gene expression of PLA2,[72] TNF-alpha,[74] NF-κB p50 precursor p105,[89] PAF-R,[69] and TLR4 in IECs.[90] PAF is an important mediator of the allergic and inflammatory response and causes systemic and mesenteric vasodilation, increased permeability, platelet aggregation, and neutrophil aggregation.[91]

Nitric Oxide

Nitric oxide (NO) is a free radical that regulates numerous physiologic as well as pathologic processes in the gastrointestinal tract. Small amounts of endogenous NO are constitutively produced in the intestine, mainly via the 2 constitutive isoforms of the enzyme NO synthase: endothelial NOS (eNOS) and neuronal NOS (nNOS). Several studies have found that eNOS is protective against intestinal inflammation in a dextran sodium sulfate colitis model.[92,93] However, using the same model, other investigators showed that eNOS and iNOS were detrimental, whereas nNOS was beneficial.[94] In normal rat small intestine, nNOS was found to suppress the gene expression of iNOS through NF-κB downregulation[95]; nNOS suppression led to IκB alpha degradation, NF-κB activation, and iNOS expression.[95] In neonatal rats, formula feeding downregulates eNOS and nNOS, whereas it upregulates iNOS[96] and in piglets, it downregulates eNOS.[97] iNOS is upregulated in a neonatal rat NEC model.[43] Intravenous infusion of L-arginine, an NO synthase substrate, attenuates intestinal injury in the neonatal piglet model of NEC, whereas L-NG-nitroarginine methyl ester, an NO synthase inhibitor, worsened the injury.[98] NO released by activated macrophages has been found to inhibit enterocyte migration.[99] The localized production of NO by villus enterocytes results in an increase in enterocyte apoptosis[100] and impaired proliferation.[101] NO mediates dendritic cell apoptosis[102] while protecting against apoptosis in other cell types.[103]

ROS

ROS are likely the final effector of PAF and many other cytokines. In the intestine, one of the main producers of ROS is the xanthine oxidase/dehydrogenase system. This enzyme is first synthetized as xanthine dehydrogenase, which catalyzes the transformation of xanthine into uric acid (xanthine + H2O + NAD→ uric acid + NADH + H+). Xanthine dehydrogenase is constitutively and abundantly expressed in the intestinal villous epithelium[104]; however, during ischemia, xanthine dehydrogenase is converted into xanthine oxidase, which not only catalyzes the transformation of xanthine into uric acid, but also leads to the production of superoxide (xanthine + H2O + O2→ Uric acid + 2O2−.+2H+). During oxidative stress, ROS leads to activation of the intestinal mitochondrial apoptotic signaling pathway[105] and IEC apoptosis via the activation of intestinal p38 MAPK.[106] In experimental NEC, intestinal ischemia has been shown to be associated with a shift from NO* to O2* production in a NOS-dependent manner.[107] Xanthine oxidase (XO) and superoxide have been shown to play a central role in intestinal reperfusion injury.[108] A central role for XO and ROS in causing intestinal injury is further supported by the protective role of allopurinol, a xanthine oxidase inhibitor, on PAF-induced bowel necrosis.[73]

Neutrophils/Macrophages

Neutrophils are thought to play an important role in NEC. Neutrophils have been shown to mediate PAF-induced bowel injury, hypotension, hemoconcentration,[109] and NF-κB activation.[19] Mice deficient in P-selectin[110] and mice treated with antibody against beta-2 integrin[111] (adhesion molecules necessary for neutrophils to roll and adhere to the endothelium) are protected against PAF-induced bowel injury. Our laboratory has found that treatment of mice with antibodies against CXCL2, a major chemokine for neutrophils, attenuated the systemic inflammation, the hypotension, and the acute intestinal injury induced by PAF.[112] However, in studies using live bacteria to induce NEC (eg, NEC induced by *Cronobacter sakazakii* infection), depletion of PMN and macrophages from the lamina propria impeded bacterial killing, decreased *C sakazakii* clearance, and exacerbated cytokine production and bowel injury.[113] In this same model, *C sakazakii* infection was shown to result in epithelial damage by recruiting dendritic cells (DCs) into the gut.[114] The interaction of DC with IECs led to increased TGF-β production, iNOS production, apoptosis, and epithelial cell damage.[114] The role of macrophages has been recently explored by other investigators who have found that prematurity is associated with a hyperinflammatory intestinal macrophage phenotype that leads to increased bowel injury.[115] These investigators showed that, during pregnancy, intestinal macrophages progressively acquire a noninflammatory profile. They found that TGF-β(2) isoform suppresses macrophage inflammatory responses in the developing intestine and protects against inflammatory mucosal injury.[115] Activated macrophages have been shown to block IEC restitution by inhibiting enterocyte gap junction via the release of nitric oxide.[99]

SYSTEMIC INFLAMMATION

In NEC, the inflammatory response is not limited to the intestine and there is evidence that the liver might play an important role in amplifying the inflammatory state.[116]

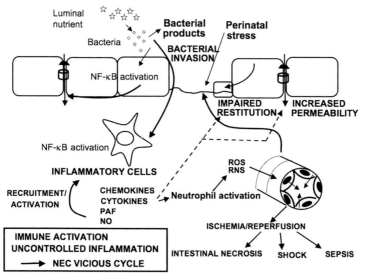

Fig. 3. Pathogenesis of NEC: current hypothesis.

Hepatic IL-18 and TNF-alpha and the number of Kupffer cells (KCs) were found to be increased in experimental NEC and to correlate with the progression of the intestinal damage.[116] TNF-alpha levels found in the intestinal lumen of rats with NEC were significantly decreased when KCs were inhibited with gadolinium chloride.[116]

SUMMARY: CURRENT HYPOTHESIS

The pathogenesis of NEC remains poorly understood (**Fig. 3**). The current but limited understanding of NEC pathogenesis is that it results from a local intestinal inflammation initiated by perinatal stress. Following the introduction of feedings, there is proliferation of intestinal bacteria, favored by the immaturity of the neonatal mucosal immune system. Intestinal bacteria and their products adhere to the epithelium, breach the immature and fragile intestinal mucosal barrier, and activate NF-κB in lamina propria immunocytes, causing them to secrete proinflammatory mediators, chemokines (CXCL2), cytokines (TNF, IL), prostanoids, PAF, and NO. (We hypothesized that the bowel injury in NEC results from inappropriately elevated and prolonged NF-κB activity in inflammatory cells.) These inflammatory agents attract further inflammatory cells, in particular neutrophils, induce the production of ROS, and inflict further damage to the intestinal barrier, resulting in increased bacterial translocation, intestinal epithelial damage, impaired epithelial cell restitution, apoptosis, and mucosal necrosis. Thus, a vicious cycle characteristic of severe NEC is created by bacterial invasion, immune activation, uncontrolled inflammation with production of ROS and nitrogen species, vasoconstriction followed by ischemia-reperfusion injury, gut barrier failure, intestinal necrosis, sepsis, and shock.

REFERENCES

1. Wang Y, Hoenig JD, Malin KJ, et al. 16S rRNA gene-based analysis of fecal microbiota from preterm infants with and without necrotizing enterocolitis. ISME J 2009;3:944–54.

2. Dinsmore JE, Jackson RJ, Smith SD. The protective role of gastric acidity in neonatal bacterial translocation. J Pediatr Surg 1997;32:1014–6.

3. Hooper LV, Wong MH, Thelin A, et al. Molecular analysis of commensal host-microbial relationships in the intestine. Science 2001;291:881–4.

4. Rozenfeld RA, Liu X, DePlaen I, et al. Role of gut flora on intestinal group II phospholipase A2 activity and intestinal injury in shock. Am J Physiol Gastrointest Liver Physiol 2001;281:G957–63.

5. Carlisle EM, Poroyko V, Caplan MS, et al. Gram negative bacteria are associated with the early stages of necrotizing enterocolitis. PLoS One 2011;6:e18084.

6. Gonzalez-Crussi F, Hsueh W. Experimental model of ischemic bowel necrosis. The role of platelet-activating factor and endotoxin. Am J Pathol 1983;112:127–35.

7. Sharma R, Tepas JJ III, Hudak ML, et al. Neonatal gut barrier and multiple organ failure: role of endotoxin and proinflammatory cytokines in sepsis and necrotizing enterocolitis. J Pediatr Surg 2007;42:454–61.

8. Essani NA, McGuire GM, Manning AM, et al. Endotoxin-induced activation of the nuclear transcription factor kappa B and expression of E-selectin messenger RNA in hepatocytes, Kupffer cells, and endothelial cells in vivo. J Immunol 1996;156:2956–63.

9. Hawiger J. Innate immunity and inflammation: a transcriptional paradigm. Immunol Res 2001;23:99–109.

10. Qu X, Huang L, Burthart T, et al. Endotoxin induces PAF production in the rat ileum: quantitation of tissue PAF by an improved method. Prostaglandin 1996;51(4):249–62.

11. Carmody RJ, Chen YH. Nuclear factor-kappaB: activation and regulation during toll-like receptor signaling. Cell Mol Immunol 2007;4:31–41.

12. Harris MC, Costarino AT Jr, Sullivan JS, et al. Cytokine elevations in critically ill infants with sepsis and necrotizing enterocolitis. J Pediatr 1994;124:105–11.

13. Viscardi RM, Lyon NH, Sun CC, et al. Inflammatory cytokine mRNAs in surgical specimens of necrotizing enterocolitis and normal newborn intestine. Pediatr Pathol Lab Med 1997;17:547–59.

14. Israel EJ, Schiffrin EJ, Carter EA, et al. Cortisone strengthens the intestinal mucosal barrier in a rodent necrotizing enterocolitis model. Adv Exp Med Biol 1991;310:375–80.

15. Claud EC, Lu L, Anton PM, et al. Developmentally regulated IkappaB expression in intestinal epithelium and susceptibility to flagellin-induced inflammation. Proc Natl Acad Sci U S A 2004;101:7404–8.

16. De Plaen IG, Liu SX, Tian R, et al. Inhibition of nuclear factor-kappaB ameliorates bowel injury and prolongs survival in a neonatal rat model of necrotizing enterocolitis. Pediatr Res 2007;61:716–21.

17. Hayden MS, Ghosh S. Signaling to NF-kappaB. Genes Dev 2004;18:2195–224.

18. Li Q, Verma IM. NF-kappaB regulation in the immune system. Nat Rev Immunol 2002;2:725–34.

19. De Plaen IG, Tan XD, Chang H, et al. Intestinal NF-kappaB is activated, mainly as p50 homodimers, by platelet-activating factor. Biochim Biophys Acta 1998;1392:185–92.

20. De Plaen IG, Tan XD, Chang H, et al. Lipopolysaccharide activates nuclear factor kappaB in rat intestine: role of endogenous platelet-activating factor and tumour necrosis factor. Br J Pharmacol 2000;129:307–14.

21. DiDonato JA, Hayakawa M, Rothwarf DM, et al. A cytokine-responsive IkappaB kinase that activates the transcription factor NF-kappaB. Nature 1997;388:548–54.

22. Minekawa R, Takeda T, Sakata M, et al. Human breast milk suppresses the transcriptional regulation of IL-1beta-induced NF-kappaB signaling in human intestinal cells. Am J Physiol Cell Physiol 2004;287:C1404–11.

23. Petrof EO, Kojima K, Ropeleski MJ, et al. Probiotics inhibit nuclear factor-kappaB and induce heat shock proteins in colonic epithelial cells through proteasome inhibition. Gastroenterology 2004;127:1474–87.

24. Chen LW, Egan L, Li ZW, et al. The two faces of IKK and NF-kappaB inhibition: prevention of systemic inflammation but increased local injury following intestinal ischemia-reperfusion. Nat Med 2003;9:575–81.

25. Egan LJ, Eckmann L, Greten FR, et al. IkappaB-kinasebeta-dependent NF-kappaB activation provides radioprotection to the intestinal epithelium. Proc Natl Acad Sci U S A 2004;101:2452–7.

26. Chae S, Eckmann L, Miyamoto Y, et al. Epithelial cell I kappa B-kinase beta has an important protective role in *Clostridium difficile* toxin A-induced mucosal injury. J Immunol 2006;177:1214–20.

27. Le Mandat Schultz A, Bonnard A, Barreau F, et al. Expression of TLR-2, TLR-4, NOD2 and pNF-kappaB in a neonatal rat model of necrotizing enterocolitis. PLoS One 2007;2:e1102.

28. De Plaen IG, Han XB, Liu X, et al. Lipopolysaccharide induces CXCL2/macrophage inflammatory protein-2 gene expression in enterocytes via NF-kappaB activation: independence from endogenous TNF-alpha and platelet-activating factor. Immunology 2006;118:153–63.

29. Shibata W, Maeda S, Hikiba Y, et al. Cutting edge: the IkappaB kinase (IKK) inhibitor, NEMO-binding domain peptide, blocks inflammatory injury in murine colitis. J Immunol 2007;179:2681–5.

30. Vancurova I, Bellani P, Davidson D. Activation of nuclear factor-kappaB and its suppression by dexamethasone in polymorphonuclear leukocytes: newborn versus adult. Pediatr Res 2001;49:257–62.

31. Kilpinen S, Henttinen T, Lahdenpohja N, et al. Signals leading to the activation of NF-kappa B transcription factor are stronger in neonatal than adult T lymphocytes. Scand J Immunol 1996;44:85–8.

32. Kelly D, Conway S. Bacterial modulation of mucosal innate immunity. Mol Immunol 2005;42:895–901.

33. Abreu MT. Toll-like receptor signalling in the intestinal epithelium: how bacterial recognition shapes intestinal function. Nat Rev Immunol 2010;10:131–44.

34. Lee J, Mo JH, Katakura K, et al. Maintenance of colonic homeostasis by distinctive apical TLR9 signalling in intestinal epithelial cells. Nat Cell Biol 2006;8:1327–36.

35. Liu Y, Zhu L, Fatheree NY, et al. Changes in intestinal Toll-like receptors and cytokines precede histological injury in a rat model of necrotizing enterocolitis. Am J Physiol Gastrointest Liver Physiol 2009;297:G442–50.

36. Gribar SC, Sodhi CP, Richardson WM, et al. Reciprocal expression and signaling of TLR4 and TLR9 in the pathogenesis and treatment of necrotizing enterocolitis. J Immunol 2009;182:636–46.

37. Tatum PM Jr, Harmon CM, Lorenz RG, et al. Toll-like receptor 4 is protective against neonatal murine ischemia-reperfusion intestinal injury. J Pediatr Surg 2010;45:1246–55.

38. Jilling T, Simon D, Lu J, et al. The roles of bacteria and TLR4 in rat and murine models of necrotizing enterocolitis. J Immunol 2006;177:3273–82.

39. Leaphart CL, Cavallo J, Gribar SC, et al. A critical role for TLR4 in the pathogenesis of necrotizing enterocolitis by modulating intestinal injury and repair. J Immunol 2007;179:4808–20.

40. Dai S, Sodhi C, Cetin S, et al. Extracellular high mobility group box-1 (HMGB1) inhibits enterocyte migration via activation of Toll-like receptor-4 and increased cell-matrix adhesiveness. J Biol Chem 2010;285:4995–5002.

41. Sodhi CP, Shi XH, Richardson WM, et al. Toll-like receptor-4 inhibits enterocyte proliferation via impaired beta-catenin signaling in necrotizing enterocolitis. Gastroenterology 2010;138:185–96.

42. Beaurepaire C, Smyth D, McKay DM. Interferon-gamma regulation of intestinal epithelial permeability. J Interferon Cytokine Res 2009;29:133–44.

43. Nadler EP, Dickinson E, Knisely A, et al. Expression of inducible nitric oxide synthase and interleukin-12 in experimental necrotizing enterocolitis. J Surg Res 2000;92:71–7.

44. Leaphart CL, Qureshi F, Cetin S, et al. Interferon-gamma inhibits intestinal restitution by preventing gap junction communication between enterocytes. Gastroenterology 2007;132:2395–411.

45. Leaphart CL, Dai S, Gribar SC, et al. Interferon-gamma inhibits enterocyte migration by reversibly displacing connexin43 from lipid rafts. Am J Physiol Gastrointest Liver Physiol 2008;295:G559–69.

46. Morecroft JA, Spitz L, Hamilton PA, et al. Plasma cytokine levels in necrotizing enterocolitis. Acta Paediatr Suppl 1994;396:18–20.

47. Edelson MB, Bagwell CE, Rozycki HJ. Circulating pro- and counterinflammatory cytokine levels and severity in necrotizing enterocolitis. Pediatrics 1999;103: 766–71.

48. Paul G, Khare V, Gasche C. Inflamed gut mucosa: downstream of interleukin-10. Eur J Clin Invest 2012;42:95–109.

49. Kuhn R, Lohler J, Rennick D, et al. Interleukin-10-deficient mice develop chronic enterocolitis. Cell 1993;75:263–74.

50. Chheda S, Palkowetz KH, Garofalo R, et al. Decreased interleukin-10 production by neonatal monocytes and T cells: relationship to decreased production and expression of tumor necrosis factor-alpha and its receptors. Pediatr Res 1996; 40:475–83.

51. Fituch CC, Palkowetz KH, Goldman AS, et al. Concentrations of IL-10 in preterm human milk and in milk from mothers of infants with necrotizing enterocolitis. Acta Paediatr 2004;93:1496–500.

52. Emami CN, Chokshi N, Wang J, et al. Role of interleukin-10 in the pathogenesis of necrotizing enterocolitis. Am J Surg 2012;203:428–35.

53. Halpern MD, Holubec H, Dominguez JA, et al. Up-regulation of IL-18 and IL-12 in the ileum of neonatal rats with necrotizing enterocolitis. Pediatr Res 2002;51: 733–9.

54. Heninger E, Treszl A, Kocsis I, et al. Genetic variants of the interleukin-18 promoter region (-607) influence the course of necrotising enterocolitis in very low birth weight neonates. Eur J Pediatr 2002;161:410–1.

55. Xu J, Treem WR, Roman C, et al. Ileal immune dysregulation in necrotizing enterocolitis: role of CD40/CD40L in the pathogenesis of disease. J Pediatr Gastroenterol Nutr 2011;52:140–6.

56. Halpern MD, Khailova L, Molla-Hosseini D, et al. Decreased development of necrotizing enterocolitis in IL-18-deficient mice. Am J Physiol Gastrointest Liver Physiol 2008;294:G20–6.

57. van Dullemen HM, van Deventer SJ, Hommes DW, et al. Treatment of Crohn's disease with anti-tumor necrosis factor chimeric monoclonal antibody (cA2). Gastroenterology 1995;109:129–35.

58. Morecroft JA, Spitz L, Hamilton PA, et al. Plasma interleukin-6 and tumour necrosis factor levels as predictors of disease severity and outcome in necrotizing enterocolitis. J Pediatr Surg 1994;29:798–800.
59. Baregamian N, Song J, Bailey CE, et al. Tumor necrosis factor-alpha and apoptosis signal-regulating kinase 1 control reactive oxygen species release, mitochondrial autophagy, and c-Jun N-terminal kinase/p38 phosphorylation during necrotizing enterocolitis. Oxid Med Cell Longev 2009;2:297–306.
60. Tan X, Hsueh W, Gonzalez-Crussi F. Cellular localization of tumor necrosis factor (TNF)-alpha transcripts in normal bowel and in necrotizing enterocolitis. TNF gene expression by Paneth cells, intestinal eosinophils, and macrophages. Am J Pathol 1993;142:1858–65.
61. Akisu M, Baka M, Yalaz M, et al. Supplementation with *Saccharomyces boulardii* ameliorates hypoxia/reoxygenation-induced necrotizing enterocolitis in young mice. Eur J Pediatr Surg 2003;13:319–23.
62. Halpern MD, Clark JA, Saunders TA, et al. Reduction of experimental necrotizing enterocolitis with anti-TNF-alpha. Am J Physiol Gastrointest Liver Physiol 2006;290:G757–64.
63. Seitz G, Warmann SW, Guglielmetti A, et al. Protective effect of tumor necrosis factor alpha antibody on experimental necrotizing enterocolitis in the rat. J Pediatr Surg 2005;40:1440–5.
64. Travadi J, Patole S, Charles A, et al. Pentoxifylline reduces the incidence and severity of necrotizing enterocolitis in a neonatal rat model. Pediatr Res 2006; 60:185–9.
65. McElroy SJ, Prince LS, Weitkamp JH, et al. Tumor necrosis factor receptor 1-dependent depletion of mucus in immature small intestine: a potential role in neonatal necrotizing enterocolitis. Am J Physiol Gastrointest Liver Physiol 2011;301:G656–66.
66. Denizot Y, Dassa E, Kim HY, et al. Synthesis of paf-acether from exogenous precursors by the prokaryote *Escherichia coli*. FEBS Lett 1989;243:13–6.
67. Denizot Y, Dassa E, Thomas Y, et al. Production of paf-acether by various bacterial strains. Gastroenterol Clin Biol 1990;14:681–2.
68. Benveniste J, Chignard M, Le Couedic JP, et al. Biosynthesis of platelet-activating factor (PAF-ACETHER). II. Involvement of phospholipase A2 in the formation of PAF-ACETHER and lyso-PAF-ACETHER from rabbit platelets. Thromb Res 1982;25:375–85.
69. Wang H, Tan X, Chang H, et al. Regulation of platelet-activating factor receptor gene expression in vivo by endotoxin, platelet-activating factor and endogenous tumour necrosis factor. Biochem J 1997;322(Pt 2):603–8.
70. Wang H, Tan X, Chang H, et al. Platelet-activating factor receptor mRNA is localized in eosinophils and epithelial cells in rat small intestine: regulation by dexamethasone and gut flora. Immunology 1999;97:447–54.
71. Lu J, Caplan MS, Li D, et al. Polyunsaturated fatty acids block platelet-activating factor-induced phosphatidylinositol 3 kinase/Akt-mediated apoptosis in intestinal epithelial cells. Am J Physiol Gastrointest Liver Physiol 2008;294:G1181–90.
72. Tan XD, Wang H, Gonzalez-Crussi FX, et al. Platelet activating factor and endotoxin increase the enzyme activity and gene expression of type II phospholipase A2 in the rat intestine. Role of polymorphonuclear leukocytes. J Immunol 1996; 156:2985–90.
73. Qu XW, Rozenfeld RA, Huang W, et al. The role of xanthine oxidase in platelet activating factor induced intestinal injury in the rat. Gut 1999;44:203–11.

74. Huang L, Tan X, Crawford SE, et al. Platelet-activating factor and endotoxin induce tumour necrosis factor gene expression in rat intestine and liver. Immunology 1994;83:65–9.

75. Caplan MS, Hedlund E, Adler L, et al. The platelet-activating factor receptor antagonist WEB 2170 prevents neonatal necrotizing enterocolitis in rats. J Pediatr Gastroenterol Nutr 1997;24:296–301.

76. Ewer AK, Al-Salti W, Coney AM, et al. The role of platelet activating factor in a neonatal piglet model of necrotising enterocolitis. Gut 2004;53:207–13.

77. Caplan MS, Lickerman M, Adler L, et al. The role of recombinant platelet-activating factor acetylhydrolase in a neonatal rat model of necrotizing enterocolitis. Pediatr Res 1997;42:779–83.

78. MacKendrick W, Hill N, Hsueh W, et al. Increase in plasma platelet-activating factor levels in enterally fed preterm infants. Biol Neonate 1993;64:89–95.

79. Caplan M, Hsueh W, Kelly A, et al. Serum PAF acetylhydrolase increases during neonatal maturation. Prostaglandins 1990;39:705–71.

80. Furukawa M, Narahara H, Yasuda K, et al. Presence of platelet-activating factor-acetylhydrolase in milk. J Lipid Res 1993;34:1603–9.

81. Muguruma K, Gray PW, Tjoelker LW, et al. The central role of PAF in necrotizing enterocolitis development. Adv Exp Med Biol 1997;407:379–82.

82. Lu J, Pierce M, Franklin A, et al. Dual roles of endogenous platelet-activating factor acetylhydrolase in a murine model of necrotizing enterocolitis. Pediatr Res 2010;68:225–30.

83. Caplan MS, Sun XM, Hsueh W. Hypoxia causes ischemic bowel necrosis in rats: the role of platelet- activating factor (PAF-acether). Gastroenterology 1990;99: 979–86.

84. Sun XM, Hsueh W. Bowel necrosis induced by tumor necrosis factor in rats is mediated by platelet-activating factor. J Clin Invest 1988;81:1328–31.

85. Hsueh W, Gonzalez-Crussi F, Arroyave JL. Platelet-activating factor: an endogenous mediator for bowel necrosis in endotoxemia. FASEB J 1987;1:403–5.

86. Hsueh W, Gonzalez-Crussi F, Arroyave JL. Platelet-activating factor-induced ischemic bowel necrosis. An investigation of secondary mediators in its pathogenesis. Am J Pathol 1986;122:231–9.

87. Caplan MS, Kelly A, Hsueh W. Endotoxin and hypoxia-induced intestinal necrosis in rats: the role of platelet activating factor. Pediatr Res 1992;31: 428–34.

88. Hsueh W, Gonzalez-Crussi F, Arroyave JL. Release of leukotriene C4 by isolated, perfused rat small intestine in response to platelet-activating factor. J Clin Invest 1986;78:108–14.

89. Tan X, Sun X, Gonzalez-Crussi FX, et al. PAF and TNF increase the precursor of NF-kappa B p50 mRNA in mouse intestine: quantitative analysis by competitive PCR. Biochim Biophys Acta 1994;1215:157–62.

90. Soliman A, Michelsen KS, Karahashi H, et al. Platelet-activating factor induces TLR4 expression in intestinal epithelial cells: implication for the pathogenesis of necrotizing enterocolitis. PLoS One 2010;5:e15044.

91. Ford-Hutchinson AW. Neutrophil aggregating properties of PAF-acether and leukotriene B4. Int J Immunopharmacol 1983;5:17–21.

92. Sasaki M, Bharwani S, Jordan P, et al. Increased disease activity in eNOS-deficient mice in experimental colitis. Free Radic Biol Med 2003;35:1679–87.

93. Vallance BA, Dijkstra G, Qiu B, et al. Relative contributions of NOS isoforms during experimental colitis: endothelial-derived NOS maintains mucosal integrity. Am J Physiol Gastrointest Liver Physiol 2004;287:G865–74.

94. Beck PL, Xavier R, Wong J, et al. Paradoxical roles of different nitric oxide synthase isoforms in colonic injury. Am J Physiol Gastrointest Liver Physiol 2004; 286:G137–47.

95. Qu XW, Wang H, De Plaen IG, et al. Neuronal nitric oxide synthase (NOS) regulates the expression of inducible NOS in rat small intestine via modulation of nuclear factor kappa B. FASEB J 2001;15:439–46.

96. D'Souza A, Fordjour L, Ahmad A, et al. Effects of probiotics, prebiotics, and synbiotics on messenger RNA expression of caveolin-1, NOS, and genes regulating oxidative stress in the terminal ileum of formula-fed neonatal rats. Pediatr Res 2010;67:526–31.

97. van Haver ER, Oste M, Thymann T, et al. Enteral feeding reduces endothelial nitric oxide synthase in the caudal intestinal microvasculature of preterm piglets. Pediatr Res 2008;63:137–42.

98. Di Lorenzo M, Bass J, Krantis A. Use of L-arginine in the treatment of experimental necrotizing enterocolitis. J Pediatr Surg 1995;30:235–40.

99. Anand RJ, Dai S, Rippel C, et al. Activated macrophages inhibit enterocyte gap junctions via the release of nitric oxide. Am J Physiol Gastrointest Liver Physiol 2008;294:G109–19.

100. Potoka DA, Upperman JS, Nadler EP, et al. NF-kappaB inhibition enhances peroxynitrite-induced enterocyte apoptosis. J Surg Res 2002;106:7–14.

101. Potoka DA, Upperman JS, Zhang XR, et al. Peroxynitrite inhibits enterocyte proliferation and modulates Src kinase activity in vitro. Am J Physiol Gastrointest Liver Physiol 2003;285:G861–9.

102. Stanford A, Chen Y, Zhang XR, et al. Nitric oxide mediates dendritic cell apoptosis by downregulating inhibitors of apoptosis proteins and upregulating effector caspase activity. Surgery 2001;130:326–32.

103. Chen Y, Stanford A, Simmons RL, et al. Nitric oxide protects thymocytes from gamma-irradiation-induced apoptosis in correlation with inhibition of p53 upregulation and mitochondrial damage. Cell Immunol 2001;214:72–80.

104. Hsueh W, Caplan MS, Qu XW, et al. Neonatal necrotizing enterocolitis: clinical considerations and pathogenetic concepts. Pediatr Dev Pathol 2003;6:6–23.

105. Baregamian N, Song J, Papaconstantinou J, et al. Intestinal mitochondrial apoptotic signaling is activated during oxidative stress. Pediatr Surg Int 2011; 27:871–7.

106. Zhou Y, Wang Q, Evers MB, et al. Oxidative stress-induced intestinal epithelial cell apoptosis is mediated by p38 MAPK. Biochem Biophys Res Commun 2006;350:860–5.

107. Whitehouse JS, Xu H, Shi Y, et al. Mesenteric nitric oxide and superoxide production in experimental necrotizing enterocolitis. J Surg Res 2010;161:1–8.

108. Parks DA, Bulkley GB, Granger DN, et al. Ischemic injury in the cat small intestine: role of superoxide radicals. Gastroenterology 1982;82:9–15.

109. Musemeche C, Caplan M, Hsueh W, et al. Experimental necrotizing enterocolitis: the role of polymorphonuclear neutrophils. J Pediatr Surg 1991;26:1047–9.

110. Sun X, Rozenfeld RA, Qu X, et al. P-selectin-deficient mice are protected from PAF-induced shock, intestinal injury, and lethality. Am J Physiol 1997;273: G56–61.

111. Sun XM, Qu XW, Huang W, et al. Role of leukocyte beta 2-integrin in PAF-induced shock and intestinal injury. Am J Physiol 1996;270:G184–90.

112. Han XB, Liu X, Hsueh W, et al. Macrophage inflammatory protein-2 mediates the bowel injury induced by platelet-activating factor. Am J Physiol Gastrointest Liver Physiol 2004;287:G1220–6.

113. Emami CN, Mittal R, Wang L, et al. Role of neutrophils and macrophages in the pathogenesis of necrotizing enterocolitis caused by *Cronobacter sakazakii*. J Surg Res 2012;172:18–28.
114. Emami CN, Mittal R, Wang L, et al. Recruitment of dendritic cells is responsible for intestinal epithelial damage in the pathogenesis of necrotizing enterocolitis by *Cronobacter sakazakii*. J Immunol 2011;186:7067–79.
115. Maheshwari A, Kelly DR, Nicola T, et al. TGF-beta2 suppresses macrophage cytokine production and mucosal inflammatory responses in the developing intestine. Gastroenterology 2011;140:242–53.
116. Halpern MD, Holubec H, Dominguez JA, et al. Hepatic inflammatory mediators contribute to intestinal damage in necrotizing enterocolitis. Am J Physiol Gastrointest Liver Physiol 2003;284:G695–702.

Newer Monitoring Techniques to Determine the Risk of Necrotizing Enterocolitis

James E. Moore, MD, PhD

KEYWORDS

- Necrotizing enterocolitis • Near-infrared spectroscopy • Monitoring technique
- Intestinal ischemia • Risk of surgery

KEY POINTS

- Necrotizing enterocolitis is a significant cause of morbidity and mortality in premature infants.
- Near-infrared spectroscopy (NIRS) can measure intestinal tissue oxygenation and detect decreases in intestinal tissue oxygenation in real time.
- Regional saturation of oxygen (rSO2) is the measurement of the tissue oxygenation level, and is dependent on the balance of the amount of O2 delivered by hemoglobin and the amount of oxygen consumed by the tissue.
- Cerebro-splanchnic oxygenation ratio (CSOR) compares splanchnic oxygenation levels with brain oxygenation values and is a way to increase the sensitivity for detection of intestinal ischemia.

INTRODUCTION

Necrotizing enterocolitis (NEC) is a devastating disease seen in the neonatal intensive care unit (NICU) and is characterized by inflammation, ischemia, and necrosis.[1] Currently up to 10% of premature infants weighing less than 1500 g are affected.[2] The overall mortality for all patients with NEC is up to 25%; however, for the one-third of patients who require surgery, that mortality can be closer to 50%.[3,4] Even as neonatal care has improved over the past 3 decades, the incidence of NEC and its associated morbidity and mortality have remained unchanged.[5]

Extensive research has revealed that NEC pathogenesis is likely multifactorial; however, both predictive and preventive strategies for this disease are lacking.[6] Because of its often-silent early progression, NEC is not always recognized until after

Disclosures: None.
Conflict of Interest: Previously was a consultant for Somanetics Corporation.
Department of Pediatrics, University of Texas, Southwestern Medical Center, 5323 Harry Hines Boulevard, Dallas, TX 75390, USA
E-mail address: james.moore@utsouthwestern.edu

Clin Perinatol 40 (2013) 125–134
http://dx.doi.org/10.1016/j.clp.2012.12.004
0095-5108/13/$ – see front matter © 2013 Elsevier Inc. All rights reserved.

clinical signs manifest. In light of its frequently fulminate progression, lack of early recognition can result in a rapid deterioration and a worse clinical outcome. The assumption is that early detection and intervention may actually lead to a reduction in mortality and morbidity, thus reducing the estimated $5 billion spent annually on this disease in the United States.[7] One current area of NEC investigation is work on developing a noninvasive means of detecting the disease in its early stages. In this review, we discuss noninvasive modalities that have shown promise in improving the early detection of NEC and focus in depth on the potential of using near infrared spectroscopy (NIRS) in this population of patients.

PATHOPHYSIOLOGY

A major problem with NEC in the preterm population is differentiating it from other common entities. Although symptoms of ileus, gastric residuals, and bowel distension are common to the diagnosis of NEC, it is also frequently seen in the presentation of spontaneous intestinal perforation, septic ileus, and feeding intolerance, as well as others. Current research suggests that although these signs and symptoms are common in very low birth weight and extremely low birth weight infants, NEC often differentiates itself by developing larger areas of intestinal inflammation and progressive elevation of serum cytokines.[8] Although the precise risk factors for NEC are not fully understood, common predisposing factors seem to be consistent. The common denominator for NEC development seems to be intestinal immaturity. This immaturity leads to issues with abnormal barrier function, absorption, intestinal microbiota composition, inflammatory response, and abnormalities in circulatory regulation.[9] These combined factors can lead to an uncontrolled inflammatory cascade that, if it progresses, will result in intestinal tissue necrosis. Understanding these risk factors and designing tests to identify these abnormalities early will hopefully lead to the development of techniques for the detection of NEC.

MONITORING TECHNIQUES FOR THE DETECTION OF NEC

Ideally, an NEC detector would have the following advantages: it would reliably identify early NEC from all other similar conditions; it would be portable, accurate, noninvasive, and easy to use; have high resolution with high sensitivity and specificity; and, in a perfect world, have a favorable cost profile. Obviously, that technology does not exist currently; however, there are current available technologies that may meet some of the conditions.

RADIOGRAPHIC IMAGING

Our current standard for detecting NEC is radiographic imaging. The concern with this method is that the identification of NEC is usually later in the course and the ability to do frequent monitoring is not possible because of concerns about radiation. The identification of pneumatosis or pneumoperitoneum demonstrates the need for medical or surgical intervention; however, at this stage of the disease process, the information is not in time to alter the clinical care to prevent intestinal damage. There are limitations associated with this technique because of the intermittent nature of the test. Conventional radiographic imaging gives you only a point in time. It therefore is possible to miss transient pneumatosis and even a small perforation. Although it is diagnostic, it is usually not early enough in the course to make a difference.

GASTRIC TONOMETRY

Gastric tonometry uses a balloon tip catheter that is inserted into the stomach. This probe measures intramucosal Pco_2 and calculates a gastric pH as an estimate for mucosal oxygenation. Previous studies have shown that intramucosal pH can be an indicator of splanchnic ischemia, systemic hypovolemia, and sepsis (presumably from changes in tissue perfusion).[10,11] Although gastric tonometry has been accepted as an indicator for splanchnic perfusion and oxygenation, its use, specifically for NEC, has yet to be fully developed.[12,13] There is evidence in a small series of patients with congenital heart disease that the decrease in gastric mucosal pH coincided with the presentation of NEC.[14]

There have been investigations into alternative sites that may be easier to obtain results, better tolerated, or more accurate. Although studies have looked at locations in the small intestine, rectum, and sublingual area, obtaining intramucosal pH at these sites still carries the disadvantage of being invasive. In addition, the rectal site was not consistent with gastric measurements.[15,16] Further, it takes up to 1.5 hours for this method to reach equilibrium; this limitation, as well as issues with changes in the test because of the presence of enteral feeds, may make this method less useful as a screening tool. Although gastric tonometry could be useful in detection of some cases of NEC, its current indication is more often for the detection of global hypoperfusion and shock. There would need to be additional studies to determine if there is an indication for NEC specifically.

SONOGRAPHY

The sonographic ability to determine pneumatosis intestinalis has been reported for more than 25 years.[17] Although early reports using ultrasound (US) were of advanced-stage disease, more recent reports have looked into detecting changes in bowel appearance in early-stage NEC.[18] The advantage of US was that it was more sensitive than plain radiographs for detecting early pneumatosis.[18] In addition, US was able to detect signs of intestinal perforation in gasless abdomens.[19]

Doppler US allows for additional information about blood flow within the mesentery. Faingold and colleagues[20] showed that color Doppler US could help determine intestinal viability by specifically looking at the perfusion to the tissue. When color Doppler failed to detect flow in the intestines, it was 100% sensitive for severe NEC and the presence of necrotic bowel. In comparison, the radiographic detection of free air was less than 50%. A major limitation to the use of US is that intraluminal air leads to artifacts, making it difficult to interpret. This would limit its usefulness in many cases of NEC.

BIOMARKERS

A number of biomarkers have been examined as predictors of NEC. Cheu and colleagues[21] examined testing for H_2 excretion. Microbial fermentation of carbohydrate results in the production of H_2 and is exhaled in the breath. They examined 122 neonates weighing less than 2000 g. They demonstrated significantly higher excretion of H_2 in infants with NEC, with a sensitivity of 86% and a specificity of 90%. The increase in H_2 concentration appeared before clinical signs of NEC; however, H_2 testing is technically difficult and its overall poor positive predictive value makes this test not as appealing for widespread use in its current form.

More recently, blood and urine sampling for different proteins has been suggested as a possible tool for the identification of markers of early NEC. Aydemir and colleagues[22] investigated whether serum intestinal fatty acid binding protein (I-FABP) levels could identify patients with NEC and predict their severity of illness. I-FABP is a water-soluble protein present in mature enterocytes and is presumably released when injured during NEC. These investigators showed a transient rise in serum I-FABP levels and their results suggested that serum I-FABP levels may be able to differentiate NEC from other gastrointestinal (GI) processes. Evennett and colleagues[23] showed that urinary I-FABP concentrations predicted extent of disease in NEC. Others have shown a potential role for the detection of enterobacterial DNA in blood management of NEC.[24] Although these markers may not be the final answer, looking for a measurable indicator protein that predicts NEC would be desirable.

Based on data from twin gestations, NEC likely has a genetic component.[25] Inflammatory and genetic markers may therefore also be candidates for identifying infants most at risk for developing NEC. Possible candidates, such as CD-14, toll-like receptor-4, interleukin-4, or others, may allow us to improve our prediction of patients who will develop NEC. A recent candidate is the single nucleotide polymorphism in carbamoyl-phosphate synthetase 1 (associated with the production of the amino acid arginine). This was recently found to be associated with increased risk of NEC development.[26] The problem currently is that most genetic markers are indicative of secondary inflammatory responses, such as sepsis, and are not acting alone. Genetic factors seem to work in conjunction with other modifiers, such as bacterial and host interactions. In addition, genetic testing is expensive and identifies only patients with potentially higher risk for NEC and therefore cannot identify patients with NEC with high specificity or sensitivity.[27]

Recent work has examined if evaluating the composition of the intestinal microbiota may be able to detect distortions in microbial patterns that may increase a patient's risk of NEC. The vast number of commensal microorganisms present in the GI track can influence physiology. This hypothesis predicts that certain microbes that are present in the host and originally contribute to the normal microflora pattern, may, after a certain set of conditions, amplify and contribute to the development of NEC.[28] The techniques for monitoring these pathogens seem promising because collection of stool is easy and noninvasive. Recent advances in 16S rRNA techniques have allowed investigators to analyze the microbiota in detail[29]; however, normal microbiota patterns in preterm infants have yet to be fully defined, and specific patterns for NEC have not yet been fully developed.[30] This topic is covered in more detail in the article by Josef Neu, elsewhere in this issue.

NEAR-INFRARED SPECTROSCOPY

Near-infrared spectroscopy (NIRS) was introduced in the 1970s. The technique was capable of noninvasively monitoring regional oxygenation in living tissue. It has been used in human studies for more than 30 years.[31] The first use in pediatrics was in sick preterm infants and examined cerebral oxygenation changes over time.[32] NIRS is a noninvasive, portable device that can continuously measure tissue oxygenation in real time.[33] The technological principle that NIRS relies on is that most biologic tissue allows near-infrared light to pass through it easily. The 2 principal compounds within human tissue that absorb light in the near-infrared range are hemoglobin and cytochrome oxidase.[34] NIRS uses light wavelengths of 700 to 1000 nm, similar to pulse oximetry, for measuring tissue oxygenation. Pulse oximetry, however, depends on pulsatile blood flow and measures only the oxygenation in arterial blood. NIRS measures the difference between oxyhemoglobin and deoxyhemoglobin, which reflects oxygen uptake in the specific tissue bed being measured.[35] This measurement is reported as the regional oxygen saturation (rSO2). NIRS measures the balance of oxygen that is delivered minus what is extracted at the tissue level. Because of the unique design of this technology, clinicians can directly monitor fluctuations in tissue oxygenation as they occur in real time. To explain this concept further, lower NIRS readings can indicate 2 possibilities: (1) increased oxygen extraction at the tissue level, or (2) decreased blood flow altering oxygen delivery to tissues in the region being measured.

NIRS AND NEC

Histologic changes in intestinal tissue from patients with NEC suggest the presence of bowel ischemia. Although NEC is a multifactorial disease, it has been hypothesized that bowel ischemia is a critical step in its development.[36] If alterations in bowel perfusion could lead to mesenteric ischemia and subsequent intestinal injury, then being able to detect tissue perfusion changes may give the clinician an earlier warning about potential disease.

Promising animal work seemed to suggest that NIRS was able to noninvasively detect changes in tissue oxygenation levels in the small bowel where blood flow was experimentally altered in real time using a piglet model.[37,38] The technology was able to detect decreased tissue oxygenation levels rapidly in the animal model, which led to the consideration of using NIRS for the detection of NEC within the human neonate.

Early reports that NIRS was able to detect changes in splanchnic oxygen delivery and predict splanchnic ischemia in neonates were reported in the literature.[39] Fortune and colleagues[39] examined splanchnic perfusion by NIRS in infants who had abdominal disease. Ten infants with acute abdomens and 29 infants admitted for other medical reasons were evaluated. Cerebral as well as splanchnic regional oxygenations were simultaneously monitored using NIRS. They determined that the ratio of cerebral to splanchnic oxygenation (cerebro-splanchnic oxygenation ratio or CSOR) was a more sensitive determinant of splanchnic ischemia, as compared with NIRS evaluation of the splanchnic bed alone. In this case, brain oxygenation was used a reference. In most physiologic conditions, cerebral blood flow autoregulation should minimize the changes in brain oxygenation during events that were specifically affecting intestinal perfusion, such as NEC. They found that if the CSOR value was less than 0.75, intestinal ischemia was identified with a positive predictive value of 0.75, and when the ratio was above 0.75, intestinal ischemia was excluded with a negative predictive value of 0.96. Five of the infants included in the study had surgical NEC, and the investigators noted that a lower ratio was identified in all 5 patients. The diagnosis of NEC was later confirmed at surgery and histology confirmed ischemic intestinal injury in all 5 patients. The investigators stressed that further evaluation of the technique was needed but its noninvasiveness and simplicity gives it exciting potential.[39]

A number of other case reports were presented that examined mesenteric oxygen desaturations that took place during the development of NEC.[40,41] These studies showed that with bowel rest and antibiotic therapy, the patients' splanchnic oxygen saturations increased as the clinical and radiographic status improved. It was proposed that changes in mesenteric NIRS might provide an early warning for developing tissue hypoxia and lead to earlier diagnosis, treatment, and perhaps even allow for the possible prevention of NEC.

LIMITATIONS OF NIRS IN MONITORING INTESTINAL TISSUE OXYGENATION IN PRETERM INFANTS

Interpretation of the rSO2 values of the mesenteric tissue bed is challenging because of the hollow structure of the intestine, peristalsis, and the large surface area. The values for tissue oxygenation in the abdomen tend to fluctuate or, simply put, are noisier than the recordings in other tissue beds. Recent studies have also demonstrated that mesenteric tissue oxygenation baselines in preterm infants first decline then slowly return to baseline over the first 7 to 14 days of life. Preterm neonates have lower starting baselines for abdominal NIRS values and the more premature the subjects, the lower their mesenteric baseline will fall during the first 2 weeks of life.[42,43] McNeil and colleagues[42] also reported that abdominal rSO_2 was the only location (vs cerebral and renal tissue beds) where values varied among gestational age groups. Although it did not reach significance, the earliest gestational age group reached an abdominal rSO_2 nadir later and had a lower rSO2 baseline value than the less premature group. These patterns suggested a possible gestational-dependent maturation in the mesenteric vasculature to provide for the increasing metabolic activity of the intestinal tract. Because it would be difficult to interpret variation versus a true decline in abdominal rSO_2 measurements around such a low baseline, the ability to detect pathologic changes during the first 2 weeks of life may be reduced. Nevertheless, the baseline for preterm neonates seems to return to expected control levels usually by 2 weeks of age. These gestational age effects on tissue oxygenation were not present in the other vascular beds examined.

Cortez and colleagues[43] also examined mesenteric tissue oxygenation in preterm infants over the first 2 weeks of life and observed that mean abdominal rSO_2 values decreased and then recovered, similar to results of McNeill and colleagues[42]; however, they also had 8 patients with feeding intolerance during this period and noted that the infants with feeding intolerance had a lower abdominal rSO_2 value compared with infants without feeding intolerance. In addition, their study had 2 infants who developed NEC, and these babies were noted to have a loss of variability and increased signal drop out, with lower baseline abdominal rSO_2 values compared with controls who did not have NEC. Additional investigation will be required to determine if abdominal pathology can be determined during the first 2 weeks of life in preterm infants.

What these two, and other unpublished studies, have established is that we cannot use term infant normative data for abdominal NIRS values during the first 2 weeks of life in the premature infant. Even though abdominal NIRS rSO_2 values remain variable (noisy) and decline in value during the early postnatal period, however, most preterm infants will return to a normal average baseline of near 60 by 2 weeks of life. Given that abdominal rSo2 values tend to recover by 2 weeks of age, NIRS may have a more important application in the preterm infant presenting after 2 weeks of age.[42] Given that premature infants at highest risk (most premature at birth) also present later in life (with presentation usually occurring at corrected gestational age of 32 weeks), NIRS may hold promise in early detection of NEC in our highest-risk infants.

SURGICAL NEC AND NIRS

Our research team has investigated whether NIRS and the direct measurement of abdominal regional saturation of oxygen (A-rSO2) could help differentiate between preterm infants with surgical NEC and preterm infants who were ill but did not have NEC. Our study examined both splanchnic perfusion changes alone, as well as changes in cerebral perfusion (the CSOR ratio). A major difference in our study, compared with the studies by McNeill and colleagues[42] and Cortez and colleagues,[43] was that all 22 study patients were more than 18 days old. This likely explains why our baseline abdominal rSO2 values in control infants were noted to be above 60 on average. Our study demonstrated that NIRS could differentiate between preterm infants with surgical NEC and infants with sepsis or another process other than an abdominal infection. Further, there appeared to be a trend, although not statistically significant, that worse preoperative abdominal NIRS values correlated with more necrotic bowel at surgery. Our results showed that 9 of 10 babies with NEC with surgically confirmed gut ischemia had a CSOR of less than 0.75. The 1 patient who had a CSOR value above 0.75 was found to have an isolated ileal perforation and appeared to be a spontaneous intestinal perforation rather than NEC. In the infants without gut ischemia present (sick controls without an abdominal focus), 0 of 12 patients had CSOR below 0.75. The NEC group had a median CSOR value of 0.54 (0.25–0.85) (P<.01). This compared with a CSOR for the sick infants without a GI process of 1.03 (0.88–1.2). Our results also support the findings by Fortune and colleagues[39] that a ratio of cerebral to somatic oxygenation may be able to predict gut ischemia. NIRS may be useful in predicting necrotic intestine when the values are low, but here we show that NIRS values may also be useful in predicting nonischemic intestinal tissue when the CSOR values are greater than 0.75. Further studies are needed to ascertain the accuracy and usefulness of NIRS in measuring splanchnic perfusion and determining if it is more accurate as a tool to rule in NEC, or actually a better tool to rule out NEC.

COULD NIRS BE USED FOR POST-NEC REFEEDING?

Although the focus of this review is discussing applications that could be used to identify NEC early in its course or identify patients who are at risk for developing NEC, we suggest that NIRS may actually have an additional application in helping determine readiness to accept feeds after NEC treatment. In an article by Dave and colleagues,[44] NIRS was used to evaluate splanchnic perfusion patterns in healthy premature infants tolerating full feeds. This group demonstrated that splanchnic tissue oxygen levels actually increase postprandially in preterm infants receiving full orogastric bolus feedings, while cerebral oxygenation levels remain unchanged.[44] Thus, CSOR values were increased following feedings in healthy preterm infants. This would make sense from a physiologic standpoint, as the body diverts blood flow to carry away digested nutrients. This likely results in more delivery of O2 (from increased blood flow), leading to an increase in tissue oxygen values measured by NIRS in the mesenteric tissue bed. Krimmel and colleagues examined Doppler US and has previously shown that superior mesenteric blood flow increases postprandially, supporting Dave and colleagues'[44,45] NIRS findings. Because the normal NIRS pattern for feeding in the healthy preterm and term infant is to have an increase in both splanchnic tissue oxygenation and increased CSOR score, it would suggest that if this response were not present that the intestinal perfusion may still be compromised after NEC. In a preliminary study, our group has looked at neonates undergoing the initiation of enteral feeds after completion of antibiotics and bowel rest for the treatment of NEC. We measured the splanchnic NIRS values and recorded the CSOR values in patients after NEC treatment. In a small group of study patients, neonates who tolerated advancing of enteral feeds had an increase in splanchnic NIRS values and an increased CSOR score, similar to what was described by Dave and colleagues.[44] In the patients who had large residuals or feeding intolerance, however, all 4 of these patients had a significant drop in mesenteric NIRS values and a fall in CSOR value sometimes to levels below 0.8. This would suggest that in these patients, the intestinal perfusion may not have normalized and that additional bowel rest is required. These results require much larger numbers to make conclusions, but the possibility of eventually being able to tailor feeding advancement to the patient's physiologic condition may allow for a more rapid return to full feeds and perhaps may reduce overall length of stay.

SUMMARY

NEC is a significant cause of morbidity and mortality in the NICU population. Although prevention strategies discussed in other articles in this issue likely will have the greatest impact in improving outcomes, detection of patients at risk for NEC and identification of the disease in its early stages remains an important challenge. NIRS currently is not the perfect NEC detector we are looking for; however, it is still a valuable tool. There are a number of methods currently available that may help identify certain cases of NEC; however, we have yet to indentify a method for the detection of NEC that is consistent, early in the course, a portable test, easy to use, sensitive, and specific. Although many of the technologies discussed in this article have potential, continued modification and discovery will have to take place to achieve our goal.

REFERENCES

1. Patel BK, Shah JS. Necrotizing enterocolitis in very low birth weight infants: a systemic review. ISRN Gastroenterol 2012;2012:562594.
2. Claud EC, Walker WA. Bacterial colonization, probiotics, and necrotizing enterocolitis. J Clin Gastroenterol 2008;42(Suppl 2):S46–52.
3. Holman RC, Stoll BJ, Curins AT, et al. Necrotising enterocolitis hospitalisations among neonates in the United States. Paediatr Perinat Epidemiol 2006;20(6): 498–506.
4. Sharma R, Hudak ML, Tepas JJ, et al. Impact of gestational age on the clinical presentation and surgical outcome of necrotizing enterocolitis. J Perinatol 2006;26(6):342–7.
5. Fitzgibbons SC, Ching Y, Yu D, et al. Mortality of necrotizing enterocolitis expressed by birth weight categories. J Pediatr Surg 2009;44(6):1072–5 [discussion: 1075–6].
6. Lin PW, Nasr TR, Stoll BJ. Necrotizing enterocolitis: recent scientific advances in pathophysiology and prevention. Semin Perinatol 2008;32(2):70–82.
7. Bisquera JA, Cooper TR, Berseth CL. Impact of necrotizing enterocolitis on length of stay and hospital charges in very low birth weight infants. Pediatrics 2002;109(3):423–8.
8. Neu J, Walker WA. Necrotizing enterocolitis. N Engl J Med 2011;364(3):255–64.
9. Lin PW, Stoll BJ. Necrotising enterocolitis. Lancet 2006;368(9543):1271–83.
10. Walley KR, Friesen BP, Humer MF, et al. Small bowel tonometry is more accurate than gastric tonometry in detecting gut ischemia. J Appl Physiol 1998;85(5):1770–7.
11. Hatherill M, Tibby SM, Evans R, et al. Gastric tonometry in septic shock. Arch Dis Child 1998;78(2):155–8.
12. Ackland G, Grocott MP, Mythen MG. Understanding gastrointestinal perfusion in critical care: so near, and yet so far. Crit Care 2000;4(5):269–81.
13. Calvo C, Ruza F, Lopez-Herce J, et al. Usefulness of gastric intramucosal pH for monitoring hemodynamic complications in critically ill children. Intensive Care Med 1997;23(12):1268–74.
14. Hatherill M, Tibby SM, Denver L, et al. Early detection of necrotizing enterocolitis by gastrointestinal tonometry. Acta Paediatr 1998;87(3):344–5.
15. Fisher EM, Kerr ME, Hoffman LA, et al. A comparison of gastric and rectal CO2 in cardiac surgery patients. Biol Res Nurs 2005;6(4):268–80.
16. Marik PE. Sublingual capnography: a clinical validation study. Chest 2001;120(3): 923–7.
17. Sigel B, Machi J, Ramos JR, et al. Ultrasonic features of pneumatosis intestinalis. J Clin Ultrasound 1985;13(9):675–8.

18. Kim WY, Kim WS, Kim IO, et al. Sonographic evaluation of neonates with early-stage necrotizing enterocolitis. Pediatr Radiol 2005;35(11):1056–61.
19. Miller SF, Seibert JJ, Kinder DL, et al. Use of ultrasound in the detection of occult bowel perforation in neonates. J Ultrasound Med 1993;12(9):531–5.
20. Faingold R, Daneman A, Tomlinson G, et al. Necrotizing enterocolitis: assessment of bowel viability with color Doppler US. Radiology 2005;235(2):587–94.
21. Cheu HW, Brown DR, Rowe MI. Breath hydrogen excretion as a screening test for the early diagnosis of necrotizing enterocolitis. Am J Dis Child 1989;143(2):156–9.
22. Aydemir C, Dilli D, Oguz SS, et al. Serum intestinal fatty acid binding protein level for early diagnosis and prediction of severity of necrotizing enterocolitis. Early Hum Dev 2011;87(10):659–61.
23. Evennett NJ, Hall NJ, Pierro A, et al. Urinary intestinal fatty acid-binding protein concentration predicts extent of disease in necrotizing enterocolitis. J Pediatr Surg 2010;45(4):735–40.
24. Mancini N, Poloniato A, Ghidoli N, et al. Potential role of the detection of enterobacterial DNA in blood for the management of neonatal necrotizing enterocolitis. J Med Microbiol 2012;61(Pt 10):1465–72.
25. Bhandari V, Bizzarro MJ, Shetty A, et al. Familial and genetic susceptibility to major neonatal morbidities in preterm twins. Pediatrics 2006;117(6):1901–6.
26. Moonen RM, Paulussen AD, Souren NY, et al. Carbamoyl phosphate synthetase polymorphisms as a risk factor for necrotizing enterocolitis. Pediatr Res 2007; 62(2):188–90.
27. Szebeni B, Szekeres R, Rusai K, et al. Genetic polymorphisms of CD14, toll-like receptor 4, and caspase-recruitment domain 15 are not associated with necrotizing enterocolitis in very low birth weight infants. J Pediatr Gastroenterol Nutr 2006;42(1):27–31.
28. Neu J. Neonatal necrotizing enterocolitis: an update. Acta Paediatr Suppl 2005; 94(449):100–5.
29. Frank DN, Pace NR. Gastrointestinal microbiology enters the metagenomics era. Curr Opin Gastroenterol 2008;24(1):4–10.
30. Peter CS, Feuerhahn M, Bohnhorst B, et al. Necrotising enterocolitis: is there a relationship to specific pathogens? Eur J Pediatr 1999;158(1):67–70.
31. Ferrari M, Giannini I, Sideri G, et al. Continuous noninvasive monitoring of human brain by near infrared spectroscopy. Adv Exp Med Biol 1985;191:873–82.
32. Brazy JE, Lewis DV, Mitnick MH, et al. Noninvasive monitoring of cerebral oxygenation in preterm infants: preliminary observations. Pediatrics 1985;75(2): 217–25.
33. Marin T, Moore J. Understanding near-infrared spectroscopy. Adv Neonatal Care 2011;11(6):382–8.
34. Wahr JA, Tremper KK, Samra S, et al. Near-infrared spectroscopy: theory and applications. J Cardiothorac Vasc Anesth 1996;10(3):406–18.
35. Chakravarti S, Srivastava S, Mittnacht AJ. Near infrared spectroscopy (NIRS) in children. Semin Cardiothorac Vasc Anesth 2008;12(1):70–9.
36. Nowicki P. Intestinal ischemia and necrotizing enterocolitis. J Pediatr 1990; 117(1 Pt 2):S14–9.
37. Gay AN, Lazar DA, Stoll B, et al. Near-infrared spectroscopy measurement of abdominal tissue oxygenation is a useful indicator of intestinal blood flow and necrotizing enterocolitis in premature piglets. J Pediatr Surg 2011;46(6):1034–40.
38. Varela JE, Cohn SM, Diaz I, et al. Splanchnic perfusion during delayed, hypotensive, or aggressive fluid resuscitation from uncontrolled hemorrhage. Shock 2003;20(5):476–80.

39. Fortune PM, Wagstaff M, Petros AJ. Cerebro-splanchnic oxygenation ratio (CSOR) using near infrared spectroscopy may be able to predict splanchnic ischaemia in neonates. Intensive Care Med 2001;27(8):1401–7.

40. Stapleton GE, Eble BK, Dickerson HA, et al. Mesenteric oxygen desaturation in an infant with congenital heart disease and necrotizing enterocolitis. Tex Heart Inst J 2007;34(4):442–4.

41. Zabaneh RN, Cleary JP, Lieber CA. Mesentric oxygen saturations in premature twins with and without necrotizing enterocolitis. Pediatr Crit Care Med 2011; 12(6):e404–6.

42. McNeill S, Gatenby JC, McElroy S, et al. Normal cerebral, renal and abdominal regional oxygen saturations using near-infrared spectroscopy in preterm infants. J Perinatol 2011;31(1):51–7.

43. Cortez J, Gupta M, Amaram A, et al. Noninvasive evaluation of splanchnic tissue oxygenation using near-infrared spectroscopy in preterm neonates. J Matern Fetal Neonatal Med 2011;24(4):574–82.

44. Dave V, Brion LP, Campbell DE, et al. Splanchnic tissue oxygenation, but not brain tissue oxygenation, increases after feeds in stable preterm neonates tolerating full bolus orogastric feeding. J Perinatol 2009;29(3):213–8.

45. Krimmel GA, Baker R, Yanowitz TD. Blood transfusion alters the superior mesenteric artery blood flow velocity response to feeding in premature infants. Am J Perinatol 2009;26(2):99–105.

The Surgical Management of Necrotizing Enterocolitis

Zachary J. Kastenberg, MD[a], Karl G. Sylvester, MD[b],*

KEYWORDS

- Necrotizing enterocolitis • Laparotomy • Primary peritoneal drainage

KEY POINTS

- Necrotizing enterocolitis (NEC) is a gastrointestinal inflammatory disease associated with prematurity.
- The optimal time to operate is when gangrenous bowel is present, but before perforation.
- The only absolute indication to operate is pneumoperitoneum on radiography.
- Operative techniques include laparotomy with bowel resection (enterostomy vs primary anastomosis), primary peritoneal drainage, "patch, drain, and wait," "clip and drop-back," and high diverting jejunostomy.
- Survival following operation is roughly 50%, and complications are common.

INTRODUCTION

Necrotizing enterocolitis (NEC) is a common cause of neonatal gastrointestinal (GI) morbidity and mortality. NEC is an inflammatory condition of the GI tract that occurs across a broad spectrum of severity, and is strongly associated with prematurity. With improved survival of premature infants, there is now a larger population at risk for developing NEC than ever before. NEC is responsible for 1% to 7% of all neonatal intensive care unit (NICU) admissions and is diagnosed in roughly 1 to 3 per 1000 live births.[1–3] The incidence increases to approximately 10% (2%–22%) in infants of very low birth weight (VLBW; ie, <1500 g).[1,4,5]

NEC is a multifactorial inflammatory disease of the GI tract. Although the exact etiology remains unknown, inciting factors often include an ischemic insult in the

---

Disclosures: None.

[a] Stanford Department of Surgery, Lucile Packard Children's Hospital, Stanford University School of Medicine, 300 Pasteur Drive, H3680D, Stanford, CA 94305-5641, USA; [b] Hagey Laboratory for Regenerative Medicine, Stanford Department of Surgery, Lucile Packard Children's Hospital, Stanford University School of Medicine, 257 Campus Drive, Stanford, CA 94305-5148, USA
* Corresponding author.
E-mail address: sylvester@stanford.edu

form of neonatal hypoxia, congenital cardiac disease, or respiratory distress syndrome, and gut colonization along with a compromised intestinal barrier function compounded by the initiation of enteral feeds. There is a higher incidence of NEC in formula-fed infants, suggesting that the immunologic and anti-inflammatory components of breast milk are protective factors.[6–9] Thus, a possible unifying theory to explain the etiology of NEC holds that an immature immune system, an underdeveloped GI mucosal barrier, and decreased bowel motility along with gut colonization conspire to produce progressive inflammation and bacterial invasion, leading to necrosis.[10–14]

Mild, nonprogressive NEC can be managed effectively through supportive care without surgery. Approximately 50% of all affected infants, however, will progress to severe disease requiring urgent surgical intervention.[15] With few absolute indications for operation and limited prospective data informing clinical decision making, there remains no consensus on the optimal approach to infants with progressive disease. An understanding of the benefits and limitations of the available diagnostic studies and surgical techniques is valuable to the practitioner who is caring for these infants.

PATIENT EVALUATION
Clinical Findings

The clinical signs of early NEC are nonspecific and overlap with those of neonatal sepsis, and can be further confused with spontaneous intestinal perforation. The earliest signs of NEC include lethargy, abdominal distention, and high gastric residuals or vomiting. Gross blood in the stool is an initial sign of disease in 25% to 63% of infants with NEC.[16,17] Clinical signs of advanced disease include vital-sign instability; abdominal wall erythema, edema, or crepitus; peritonitis; a palpable abdominal mass; or, occasionally, a discolored scrotum suggestive of bowel perforation.

Laboratory Investigations

The laboratory findings typical of NEC are nonspecific, but in conjunction with the appropriate clinical and radiographic signs can be highly suggestive of the disease. Commonly seen is the triad of neutropenia, thrombocytopenia, and metabolic acidosis. One study reported an absolute neutrophil count of fewer than 1500 cells/mm^3 to be present in 37% of infants with NEC.[18] In addition, those infants with lower neutrophil counts had worse outcomes. Thrombocytopenia is a sensitive, but nonspecific, marker of NEC found in 65% to 90% of affected infants.[18,19] Metabolic acidosis is also a nonspecific finding, but likely reflects the consequences of both intestinal and systemic hypoperfusion. In addition to these basic hematologic studies, both plasma C-reactive protein and stool-reducing substances often aid in the diagnosis of NEC. Unfortunately, no combination of laboratory results is specific enough to confirm the diagnosis of NEC or to serve as an absolute indication for surgical intervention.

Radiographic Studies

Two-view abdominal radiography (supine and left lateral decubitus) provides the classic diagnostic signs of NEC (**Fig. 1**). Generalized intestinal dilatation consistent with ileus is observed in nearly 100% of infants with NEC, and is typically present early in the disease process.[20] In the appropriate clinical setting pneumatosis intestinalis is considered pathopneumonic, but is notoriously fleeting and can be absent in up to 14% of those with severe disease (see **Fig. 1A**).[21] Portal venous gas is an ominous sign of advanced disease associated with poor outcomes, and is seen on radiography

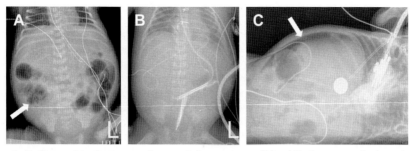

Fig. 1. Radiographic features of necrotizing enterocolitis. (*A*) Pneumatosis intestinalis (*arrow*). (*B*) Whiteout of the abdomen suggesting perforated bowel with ascites. (*C*) Pneumoperitoneum (*arrow*).

in approximately 10% to 30% of infants with NEC.[21–23] Ascites manifests as either centrally dilated loops of bowel surrounded by peripheral opacification ("floating bowel") or as a gasless, distended abdomen, and is suggestive of perforation (see **Fig. 1**B). Free air on a lateral decubitus film or the "football sign" (outlining of the falciform ligament) on a supine radiograph also indicates perforation (see **Fig. 1**C). However, only approximately 60% of infants with confirmed perforation at operation will have free air on preoperative imaging.[24]

Upper GI contrast studies may be useful in confirming the diagnosis of NEC, but are not recommended in the acute setting. Contrast gastrointestinal studies are more commonly obtained to identify intestinal strictures after the resolution of the acute illness. In the acute setting, findings suggestive of NEC include thickened bowel wall, irregular intestinal mucosa, or pneumatosis intestinalis. Care should be taken to avoid barium contrast in infants with suspected NEC, given the risk of barium peritonitis if perforation is present. Contrast enemas should be avoided in the setting of acute disease, given the risk of rectosigmoid perforation and the limited ability to identify disease proximal to the ileocecal valve.

Ultrasonography (US) has emerged as an adjunctive radiographic technique used occasionally in the diagnosis of NEC. The main utility of US is its ability to identify and localize intra-abdominal fluid for paracentesis. It may also be used to delineate portal venous gas, pneumatosis intestinalis, thinning of the bowel wall, or decreased bowel perfusion.[25] In 2005 Faingold and colleagues[26] reported the superior ability of US (relative to abdominal radiography) in diagnosing bowel necrosis in infants with suspected NEC based on Doppler-identified areas of bowel hypoperfusion. The utility of US was again supported by a 2011 study showing a combined diagnostic sensitivity of 89% for NEC when both portal venous gas on US and pneumatosis intestinalis on abdominal radiography were present, compared with sensitivities of 82% and 75% when these 2 modalities were used independently.[27] Unfortunately, this technology continues to be limited by interobserver variability and availability of on-site technologists.

Paracentesis

Paracentesis is an adjunctive study performed when clinical suspicion for intestinal gangrene or perforation is high but when confirmatory laboratory or radiographic findings are lacking. There currently exist no absolute indications for paracentesis. Paracentesis is performed at the bedside with the infant in the partial lateral decubitus position. Needle aspiration is performed under local anesthesia. A positive test is defined as more than 0.5 mL of free-flowing brown or yellow fluid containing bacteria on Gram stain.

CLASSIFICATION

In 1978, Bell and colleagues[28] proposed a set of clinical and radiographic criteria that divides infants into 1 of 3 stages of disease: stage I, suspected disease; stage II, confirmed disease without need for surgical intervention; stage III, gangrenous bowel requiring operation. Bell's criteria were modified to include substages in 1987, and continue to be used today to guide initial clinical management (**Table 1**).[29] These criteria, however, have limited ability to predict which infants with mild disease will progress to require an operation. This lack of prognostic ability leads to close NICU monitoring and serial laboratory and radiographic investigations for all infants with stage I or stage II disease. Such (currently necessary) inefficiencies support the need for the incorporation of advanced diagnostic and prognostic tools into the clinical algorithm for managing infants with NEC (**Fig. 2**).

NONOPERATIVE MANAGEMENT

Infants with Bell stage I or II are managed initially without operation. Treatment consists of cessation of enteral feedings, sump-tube gastric decompression, empiric antibiotic coverage, and frequent clinical examinations. In addition, serial 2-view abdominal radiography and laboratory tests (chemistries, complete blood count, and arterial blood gas) are obtained every 6 to 8 hours. Antibiotic choice depends on the local nursery flora and hospital antibiograms, but typically consists of a penicillin (ampicillin), an aminoglycoside (gentamicin), and an agent with anaerobic coverage (metronidazole). The increasing prevalence of resistant strains of coagulase-negative staphylococci have led some to treat empirically with vancomycin in place of a more traditional penicillin derivative. In the absence of progression to stage III disease, antibiotics are continued for 7 to 14 days and total parenteral nutrition (TPN) is initiated. Enteric nutrition is resumed slowly as gastric-tube output decreases. Stool is tested for occult blood and reducing substances after initiation of enteral feeds, either of which, if present, should prompt a return to bowel rest.

OPERATIVE MANAGEMENT
Indications for Operation

In the setting of progressive NEC, the goal of operative management is to remove gangrenous bowel while preserving intestinal length. Operation is ideally undertaken when gangrenous bowel is present but when perforation has not yet occurred. Unfortunately, there exists no combination of clinical signs, laboratory values, or radiographic findings with the ability to reliably identify this window of opportunity.

Pneumoperitoneum is the only widely accepted absolute indication for operation. Unfortunately, this finding presents only after perforation has occurred and, as previously stated, is present in only approximately 60% of those with confirmed perforation at operation.[24] Relative indications for operation include continued clinical deterioration despite optimal medical management, portal venous gas (PVG), ascites, positive paracentesis, fixed intestinal loop (same appearance of a dilated loop of bowel on radiography over 24 hours), abdominal tenderness on examination, abdominal wall erythema, and progressive thrombocytopenia.

Kosloske[30] studied 147 infants with NEC in an attempt to identify the strongest preoperative predictors of intestinal gangrene. Pneumoperitoneum, PVG, and positive paracentesis were described as "best indicators," with positive predictive values of nearly 100% and prevalence of greater than 10% in the studied population. Fixed intestinal loop, abdominal wall erythema, and palpable abdominal mass also had

Table 1
Modified Bell staging criteria for necrotizing enterocolitis

Stage	Systemic Signs	Abdominal Signs	Radiographic Signs
IA: Suspected	Temperature instability, apnea, bradycardia, lethargy	Gastric retention, abdominal distention, emesis, heme-positive stool	Normal or intestinal dilatation, mild ileus
IB: Suspected	Same as above	Same as above, plus grossly bloody stool	Same as above
IIA: Confirmed NEC (mild disease)	Same as above	Same as above, plus absent bowel sounds with or without abdominal tenderness	Intestinal dilatation, ileus, pneumatosis intestinalis
IIB: Confirmed NEC (moderate disease)	Same as above, plus mild metabolic acidosis and thrombocytopenia	Same as above, with or without abdominal cellulitis or right lower quadrant mass	Same as above, plus ascites, with or without portal vein gas
IIIA: Advanced NEC (bowel intact)	Same as above, plus hypotension, bradycardia, severe apnea, combined respiratory and metabolic acidosis, disseminated intravascular coagulation, and neutropenia	Same as above, plus signs of peritonitis, marked tenderness, and abdominal distention	Same as above
IIIB: Advanced NEC (perforated bowel)	Same as above	Same as above	Same as above, plus pneumoperitoneum

Adapted from Kliegman RM, Walsh MC. Neonatal necrotizing enterocolitis: pathogenesis, classification, and spectrum of illness. Curr Probl Pediatr 1987;17(4):213–88.

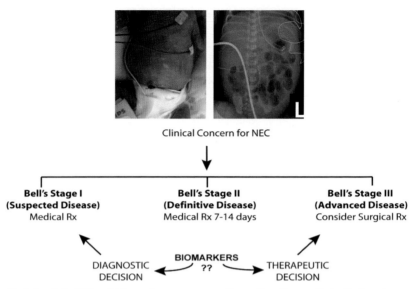

Clinical Concern for NEC

| Bell's Stage I (Suspected Disease) Medical Rx | Bell's Stage II (Definitive Disease) Medical Rx 7-14 days | Bell's Stage III (Advanced Disease) Consider Surgical Rx |

DIAGNOSTIC DECISION ← **BIOMARKERS** ?? → THERAPEUTIC DECISION

Fig. 2. Potential utility of biomarkers as prognostic and/or diagnostic indicators in necrotizing enterocolitis.

positive predictive values of 100%, but were present in less than 10% of the population and were thus termed "good indicators." Severe pneumatosis (defined as focal pneumatosis in 4 quadrants or diffuse pneumatosis) had a positive predictive value of 94% and was termed a "fair indicator." Of importance is that none of these indicators had a sensitivity of greater than 48%.

Laparotomy

The standard operation performed for necrotizing enterocolitis is laparotomy with resection of gangrenous bowel and enterostomy formation. This procedure adheres to the most basic principles of abdominal surgery: removal of necrotic tissue, diversion of proximal luminal flow, and avoidance of anastomosis in the setting of active infection or contamination. High stomal complication rates along with the need to preserve bowel length, however, have led to the development of novel techniques that challenge these principles. Reports have been published in recent decades describing the use of resection with primary anastomosis,[31–34] proximal jejunostomy without resection,[35–37] the "patch, drain, and wait" technique,[38,39] and the "clip and drop-back" technique (**Table 2**).[40] Deciding which operation to perform often depends on the personal experience of the surgeon and the extent of disease found at exploration: focal, multisegmental, or panintestinal.

Focal disease is defined as a single section of gangrenous bowel involving less than 25% of the total bowel length, and is found at laparotomy in 30% of infants with NEC.[34] The standard operation performed in this setting is resection with enterostomy formation. Laparotomy is performed through a transverse supraumbilical incision. The affected bowel is resected with creation of a proximal diverting ostomy and distal mucus fistula. The stomas can be exteriorized through the laparotomy incision, or if inflammatory mesenteric tethering prohibits this, a new incision is created for stoma creation. The bowel is typically secured to the fascia with interrupted sutures, and no attempt is made to "mature" the stoma. Restoration of bowel continuity is

Table 2
Surgical approaches for necrotizing enterocolitis

Approach	Relevant Evidence	Current Use
Bowel resection with enterostomy	For: Randomized controlled trials showing short-term outcomes equivalent to peritoneal drainage[50,51] Preliminary studies suggesting improved neurodevelopmental outcomes compared with primary peritoneal drainage[64] Against: High peristomal complication rates[42]	Standard of care when primary anastomosis is infeasible
Bowel resection with primary anastomosis	For: Avoidance of peristomal complications Improved survival in retrospective studies[32,34] Against: Prospective studies, controlling for selection bias needed before use in nonideal settings	Used in the setting of (1) focal disease, (2) viable remaining intestine, and (3) stable overall physiology
High jejunostomy	For: Case reports/series describing success in multisegmental or panintestinal NEC[35–37] Against: Prolonged dependence on total parenteral nutrition[37] High peristomal complication rates[42]	Used sparingly in multisegmental or pan-intestinal disease when initial resection would result in short-bowel syndrome
Clip and drop-back	For: Case series describing utility in infants with extensive NEC[40,65] Against: Lack of prospective evidence comparing this technique to laparotomy with enterostomy formation	Used sparingly
Patch, drain, and wait	For: Case series describing utility in infants with extensive NEC[38,39] Against: Lack of prospective evidence comparing this technique to laparotomy with enterostomy formation	Used sparingly
Primary peritoneal drainage	For: Randomized controlled trials showing short-term outcomes equivalent to laparotomy[50,51] Decreased invasiveness Against: Preliminary studies suggesting poorer neurodevelopmental outcomes when compared with laparotomy[64] As few as 11% of patients undergoing primary peritoneal drainage are managed successfully without requiring future laparotomy[51]	Ongoing debate regarding utility and long-term outcomes. Used when infant too unstable to undergo laparotomy

performed 4 to 8 weeks following resolution, depending on the severity and extent of the acute disease.

Unfortunately, 23% to 34% of infants with enterostomies will have stoma-related complications including skin excoriation; stoma stricture, retraction, or prolapse; peristomal hernia; wound infection, dehiscence, or fistula; and prolonged TPN dependence.[41,42] Resection with primary anastomosis avoids these stoma-related complications and is becoming more widely accepted as an initial operative technique in select clinical situations. Although no randomized controlled trials exist, retrospective studies report 76% to 85% overall survival following resection with primary anastomosis in comparison with 39% to 50% survival following resection with enterostomy.[32,34] While awaiting more rigorous evidence, surgical principles and surgeon experience would suggest that primary anastomosis is best suited for infants meeting the following criteria: (1) a sharply localized segment of disease, (2) healthy remaining intestine, and (3) stable overall physiology.

Multisegmental disease is found in approximately 55% of infants with NEC requiring an operation, and is defined as multiple discontinuous segments of affected bowel involving less than 50% of the total bowel length.[34] The standard operation for multisegmental disease is resection of all affected segments with multiple enterostomy formation. Primary anastomosis with avoidance of enterostomy complications has been gaining traction for multifocal disease,[34] but should still be limited to those infants meeting the aforementioned criteria. High proximal diversion termed, high jejunostomy, has been used with success in multifocal disease[35] but is associated with prolonged TPN requirements, electrolyte abnormalities, and peristomal skin complications.

In 1989, Moore[38] introduced a novel approach to infants with severe, multisegmental NEC termed the patch, drain, and wait technique. The key features of this technique are suture approximation of any perforations without resection, peritoneal drainage to the bilateral lower quadrants, placement of a gastrostomy tube, and acceptance of the need for prolonged TPN. A subsequent follow-up study reported 0% 60-day mortality in 23 infants managed with this technique.[39] Moore acknowledges that the "patch" aspect of the procedure is the least critical maneuver,[39] thus addressing concerns over the inability of gangrenous bowel to hold sutures; however, with the increased use of primary peritoneal drainage (described later), few have adopted the patch, drain, and wait technique.

In 1996, Vaughan and colleagues[40] introduced the clip and drop-back technique for use in situations where resection of all marginally viable bowel would result in short-bowel syndrome. This technique involves resection of necrotic bowel with surgical clipping (12-mm titanium clips or 35-mm autostapling device) of the bowel ends. All remaining bowel is returned to the peritoneal cavity, which is then copiously irrigated and closed. A second-look laparotomy is performed at 48 to 72 hours, at which point any necrotic bowel is removed and continuity is restored. If bowel of marginal viability remains, the clip and drop-back procedure is repeated followed by a third-look laparotomy. With initially promising results, this technique is currently used sparingly.

Panintestinal NEC, defined as less than 25% viable bowel, occurs in 15% of infants undergoing laparotomy and presents a highly controversial scenario.[34] Treatment options include resection of all necrotic bowel with multiple enterostomy formation, accepting the very high likelihood of TPN dependence if the infant survives; proximal jejunostomy with a planned second-look procedure; the patch, drain, and wait procedure; or the clip and drop-back procedure. The open-and-close laparotomy—deciding to forgo any treatment—is supported by the near 100% mortality rate associated with panintestinal NEC and the high incidence of short-bowel syndrome in survivors.[43,44]

Primary Peritoneal Drainage

Primary peritoneal drainage (PPD), an alternative to laparotomy in certain situations, is performed at the bedside under local anesthesia. A small incision is made in the right lower quadrant and the abdomen is entered under direct visualization; stool and air are often expressed on entry into the peritoneal cavity. A 0.25-inch (6.35-mm) Penrose drain is then directed to the right upper quadrant and sutured to the skin. A second drain may be placed in the left lower quadrant. The drains allow capture of fecal effluent, and fistula formation or physiologic stabilization for intestinal recovery. This technique was first described by Ein and colleagues[45] in 1977 as a means to temporize infants with NEC who were too unstable to undergo laparotomy. Subsequent reports described PPD as a definitive therapy, avoiding laparotomy and bowel resection altogether.[46–49] Until recently, however, no randomized trials that compared PPD with laparotomy were conducted.

In 2006, Moss and colleagues[50] reported the results of a multicenter, randomized controlled trial comparing PPD with laparotomy in 117 VLBW (<1500 g) infants with intestinal perforation secondary to NEC. The investigators found no difference in 90-day mortality (34.5% vs 35.5%; $P = .92$), 90-day TPN dependence (47.2% vs 40.0%; $P = .53$), or mean length of hospital stay (126 ± 58 vs 116 ± 56 days; $P = .43$). Subgroup analysis revealed no difference in mortality or TPN dependence between treatment groups for infants weighing less than 1000 g or with blood pH less than 7.30, arguing against the belief that PPD was superior to laparotomy in smaller, sicker infants. This trial, though groundbreaking and methodologically superior to prior reports, did not reach its enrollment goal of 130 patients and thus was able only to detect a reduction in mortality from 50% to 25% at 0.77 power.

A second randomized controlled trial comparing PPD with laparotomy was reported by Rees and colleagues[51] in 2008. Sixty-nine infants of extremely low birth weight (ELBW) (<1000 g) with pneumoperitoneum on radiography were enrolled. In agreement with the previous trial, Rees and colleagues found no difference in 1-month mortality (34.3% vs 24.2%; $P = .4$) or 6-month mortality (48.6% vs 36.4%; $P = .3$) between PPD and laparotomy, respectively; they also reported a 74% rate of delayed laparotomy at a median of 2.5 days following peritoneal drainage. After excluding early mortalities, only 11% of the infants in the PPD group were ultimately managed successfully without laparotomy. In the analysis of secondary outcomes, there was no difference between groups with respect to length of stay in hospital, days of ventilator dependence, TPN dependence, or days to full enteral feeds. In light of these results, Rees and colleagues concluded that early laparotomy was desirable, and that in the setting of PPD a timely "rescue" laparotomy should be performed.

COMPLICATIONS AND LONG-TERM OUTCOMES
Intestinal Stricture

Intestinal strictures develop in 9% to 36% of all patients with NEC, and are more common following nonoperative management.[52,53] In contrast to acute NEC, which most commonly affects the terminal ileum/cecum, the most common site of post-NEC stricture is the left colon (80%), with a predilection for the vascular watershed region of the splenic flexure.[54] The terminal ileum (15%) is the next most common location for post-NEC stricture. Strictures typically manifest as failure to thrive, obstructive symptoms, or rectal bleeding. These signs should prompt both an upper GI contrast study with small bowel follow-through and a barium enema. The typical management following diagnosis of an intestinal stricture is elective resection with anastomosis.

Recurrent Necrotizing Enterocolitis

Recurrent NEC has an incidence of 4% to 6%.[44,55] Episodes of recurrent NEC occur at a median of 37 days following the initial onset, and there is no clear association with timing of enteral feeding, anatomic location of initial disease, or method (operative or nonoperative) of initial management.[55] Approximately 70% of recurrent cases are successfully managed nonoperatively.

Short-Bowel Syndrome

Short-bowel syndrome is characterized by chronic malnutrition secondary to insufficient mucosal absorptive area. A general rule of thumb is that greater than 30 cm of bowel with intact ileocecal valve or greater than 50 cm of bowel without the ileocecal valve is required for an infant to survive on enteral nutrition alone. When this length of salvageable bowel is not present the short-bowel syndrome ensues, leaving the infant TPN dependent. This long-term GI complication is the most serious complication of NEC, and occurs in up to 23% of NEC survivors who required an operation.[56]

Cholestatic Liver Disease

Cholestatic liver disease occurs in the setting of prolonged TPN and is characterized by direct hyperbilirubinemia, transaminase elevation, and hepatomegaly. Treatment consists of limiting TPN use to the shortest duration possible and instituting trophic enteral feeds as early as possible. Trophic enteral nutrition aids in the recovery of mucosal health and remodeling, in addition to stimulating bile excretion.

Anastomotic (Marginal) Ulcer

Anastomotic ulcer formation is a late complication of NEC. In a series of 6 patients with post-NEC anastomotic ulcer the patients ranged in age from 5 to 13 years, and all 6 had undergone neonatal resection of the terminal ileum, ileocecal valve, and proximal colon.[57] Diagnosis was by colonoscopy, and treatment required resection and reanastomosis. The etiology of the ulceration and the true incidence of this complication are unknown.

Neurodevelopmental Impairment

Deficits in neurodevelopment are common in the premature population, and are related to a combination of medical and social factors associated with prolonged neonatal hospitalization. Historically the high incidence of neurodevelopmental delay found in NEC survivors was attributed to the high rates of prematurity in the NEC population. Recent studies, however, have challenged this belief. A study of 1151 ELBW (<1000 g) survivors at 18 to 22 months' corrected age found NEC to be an independent risk factor for both an abnormal neurologic examination and a low Bayley Psychomotor Development Index.[58] A subsequent analysis of VLBW (<1500 g) infants with NEC matched to a cohort of infants without NEC at 20 months' corrected age found incidence of severe psychomotor disability of 55% in the NEC cohort compared with 22.5% in the non-NEC control group ($P = .01$).[59]

Of interest, a study of 2948 patients in the National Institute of Child Health and Human Development (NICHD) Neonatal Research Network Registry found NEC requiring an operation (ie, surgical NEC) to be a significant independent risk factor for Mental Developmental Index less than 70 (odds ratio [OR]: 1.61; 95% confidence interval [CI]: 1.05–2.50), Psychomotor Developmental Index less than 70 (OR: 1.95; 95% CI: 1.25–3.04), and neurodevelopmental impairment (OR: 1.78; 95% CI: 1.17–2.73) when compared with NEC managed nonoperatively.[60] These findings were subsequently supported by the results of 2 systematic reviews, both showing increased odds of neurodevelopmental impairment in infants with surgical NEC relative to those with NEC managed medically.[61,62]

Such results suggest that not only the diagnosis of NEC but also the severity of the disease and the presence of circulating inflammatory mediators may contribute to the ultimate neurodevelopmental outcome. This theory is supported by a study showing increased odds of diparetic cerebral palsy in infants with both surgical NEC and late bacteremia (OR: 8.4; 95% CI: 1.9–39) in comparison with those with surgical NEC without late bacteremia (OR: 1.3; 95% CI: 0.1–11) when using premature infants with neither surgical NEC nor late bacteremia as baseline.[63]

In addition to assessing neurodevelopmental outcomes relative to the severity of the acute inflammatory process, research has been aimed at identifying differences in long-term outcomes based on the type of surgical procedure performed. In 2006 Blakely and colleagues[64] reported an intriguing disparity in neurodevelopmental outcomes when comparing initial laparotomy with peritoneal drainage. The investigators studied 156 patients with either NEC (n = 96, 62%) or intestinal perforation (n = 60, 38%), of whom 76 had initial laparotomy and 80 had initial peritoneal drainage. At 18 to 22 months' corrected age, 68% (48 of 76) in the laparotomy group were either dead or had developed neurodevelopmental impairment compared with 84% (64 of 80) in the peritoneal drainage group. These results failed to reach statistical significance after correcting for severity of illness, but still trended toward worse outcomes in the peritoneal drainage group. The NICHD Neonatal Research Network subsequently designed a follow-up randomized trial comparing laparotomy with peritoneal drainage for infants with NEC to further assess mid-term to long-term outcomes. It is anticipated that the results of this study, which at present are forthcoming, will further enlighten the debate surrounding the appropriate initial surgical management for infants with severe NEC.

SUMMARY

NEC is a common and debilitating disease of infancy. Despite the introduction of numerous novel surgical techniques, no single optimal strategy exists for the management of this complex and variable pathologic condition. Further prospective trials are needed to evaluate the existing operative approaches, and measurable improvements in both short-term and long-term outcomes will likely depend on the continued development of improved prognostic tools and preventive therapies.

REFERENCES

1. Guthrie SO, Gordon PV, Thomas V, et al. Necrotizing enterocolitis among neonates in the United States. J Perinatol 2003;23(4):278–85.
2. Hallstrom M, Koivisto AM, Janas M, et al. Frequency of and risk factors for necrotizing enterocolitis in infants born before 33 weeks of gestation. Acta Paediatr 2003;92(1):111–3.
3. Kosloske AM. Epidemiology of necrotizing enterocolitis. Acta Paediatr 1994;396: 2–7.
4. Kamitsuka MD, Horton MK, Williams MA. The incidence of necrotizing enterocolitis after introducing standardized feeding schedules for infants between 1250 and 2500 grams and less than 35 weeks of gestation. Pediatrics 2000;105(2): 379–84.
5. Lemons JA, Bauer CR, Oh W, et al. Very low birth weight outcomes of the National Institute of Child Health and Human Development Neonatal Research Network,

January 1995 through December 1996. NICHD Neonatal Research Network. Pediatrics 2001;107(1):E1.

6. Buescher ES. Host defense mechanisms of human milk and their relations to enteric infections and necrotizing enterocolitis. Clin Perinatol 1994;21(2):247–62.

7. Caplan MS, Amer M, Jilling T. The role of human milk in necrotizing enterocolitis. Adv Exp Med Biol 2002;503:83–90.

8. Goldman AS, Thorpe LW, Goldblum RM, et al. Anti-inflammatory properties of human milk. Acta Paediatr Scand 1986;75(5):689–95.

9. Hamosh M. Bioactive factors in human milk. Pediatr Clin North Am 2001;48(1):69–86.

10. Bates MD. Development of the enteric nervous system. Clin Perinatol 2002;29(1): 97–114.

11. Berseth CL. Gestational evolution of small intestine motility in preterm and term infants. J Pediatr 1989;115(4):646–51.

12. Pang KY, Bresson JL, Walker WA. Development of the gastrointestinal mucosal barrier. Evidence for structural differences in microvillus membranes from newborn and adult rabbits. Biochim Biophys Acta 1983;727(1):201–8.

13. Uauy RD, Fanaroff AA, Korones SB, et al. Necrotizing enterocolitis in very low birth weight infants: biodemographic and clinical correlates. National Institute of Child Health and Human Development Neonatal Research Network. J Pediatr 1991;119(4):630–8.

14. Udall JN, Pang K, Fritze L, et al. Development of gastrointestinal mucosal barrier. I. The effect of age on intestinal permeability to macromolecules. Pediatr Res 1981;15(3):241–4.

15. Kosloske AM. Surgery of necrotizing enterocolitis. World J Surg 1985;9(2):277–84.

16. Kanto WP Jr, Hunter JE, Stoll BJ. Recognition and medical management of necrotizing enterocolitis. Clin Perinatol 1994;21(2):335–46.

17. Chandler JC, Hebra A. Necrotizing enterocolitis in infants with very low birth weight. Semin Pediatr Surg 2000;9(2):63–72.

18. Hutter JJ Jr, Hathaway WE, Wayne ER. Hematologic abnormalities in severe neonatal necrotizing enterocolitis. J Pediatr 1976;88(6):1026–31.

19. Sola MC, Del Vecchio A, Rimsza LM. Evaluation and treatment of thrombocytopenia in the neonatal intensive care unit. Clin Perinatol 2000;27(3):655–79.

20. Daneman A, Woodward S, de Silva M. The radiology of neonatal necrotizing enterocolitis (NEC). A review of 47 cases and the literature. Pediatr Radiol 1978;7(2):70–7.

21. Kliegman RM, Fanaroff AA. Neonatal necrotizing enterocolitis in the absence of pneumatosis intestinalis. Am J Dis Child 1982;136(7):618–20.

22. Buonomo C. The radiology of necrotizing enterocolitis. Radiol Clin North Am 1999;37(6):1187–98, vii.

23. Molik KA, West KW, Rescorla FJ, et al. Portal venous air: the poor prognosis persists. J Pediatr Surg 2001;36(8):1143–5.

24. Frey EE, Smith W, Franken EA Jr, et al. Analysis of bowel perforation in necrotizing enterocolitis. Pediatr Radiol 1987;17(5):380–2.

25. Epelman M, Daneman A, Navarro OM, et al. Necrotizing enterocolitis: review of state-of-the-art imaging findings with pathologic correlation. Radiographics 2007;27(2):285–305.

26. Faingold R, Daneman A, Tomlinson G, et al. Necrotizing enterocolitis: assessment of bowel viability with color Doppler US. Radiology 2005;235(2):587–94.

27. Bohnhorst B, Kuebler JF, Rau G, et al. Portal venous gas detected by ultrasound differentiates surgical NEC from other acquired neonatal intestinal diseases. Eur J Pediatr Surg 2011;21(1):12–7.

28. Bell MJ, Ternberg JL, Feigin RD, et al. Neonatal necrotizing enterocolitis. Therapeutic decisions based upon clinical staging. Ann Surg 1978;187(1):1–7.
29. Kliegman RM, Walsh MC. Neonatal necrotizing enterocolitis: pathogenesis, classification, and spectrum of illness. Curr Probl Pediatr 1987;17(4):213–88.
30. Kosloske AM. Indications for operation in necrotizing enterocolitis revisited. J Pediatr Surg 1994;29(5):663–6.
31. Harberg FJ, McGill CW, Saleem MM, et al. Resection with primary anastomosis for necrotizing enterocolitis. J Pediatr Surg 1983;18(6):743–6.
32. Griffiths DM, Forbes DA, Pemberton PJ, et al. Primary anastomosis for necrotising enterocolitis: a 12-year experience. J Pediatr Surg 1989;24(6):515–8.
33. Ade-Ajayi N, Kiely E, Drake D, et al. Resection and primary anastomosis in necrotizing enterocolitis. J R Soc Med 1996;89(7):385–8.
34. Fasoli L, Turi RA, Spitz L, et al. Necrotizing enterocolitis: extent of disease and surgical treatment. J Pediatr Surg 1999;34(7):1096–9.
35. Martin LW, Neblett WW. Early operation with intestinal diversion for necrotizing enterocolitis. J Pediatr Surg 1981;16(3):252–5.
36. Firor HV. Use of high jejunostomy in extensive NEC. J Pediatr Surg 1982;17(6): 771–2.
37. Sugarman ID, Kiely EM. Is there a role for high jejunostomy in the management of severe necrotising enterocolitis? Pediatr Surg Int 2001;17(2–3):122–4.
38. Moore TC. The management of necrotizing enterocolitis. Pediatr Surg Int 1989;4: 110–3.
39. Moore TC. Successful use of the "patch, drain, and wait" laparotomy approach to perforated necrotizing enterocolitis: is hypoxia-triggered "good angiogenesis" involved? Pediatr Surg Int 2000;16(5–6):356–63.
40. Vaughan WG, Grosfeld JL, West K, et al. Avoidance of stomas and delayed anastomosis for bowel necrosis: the 'clip and drop-back' technique. J Pediatr Surg 1996;31(4):542–5.
41. Musemeche CA, Kosloske AM, Ricketts RR. Enterostomy in necrotizing enterocolitis: an analysis of techniques and timing of closure. J Pediatr Surg 1987;22(6): 479–83.
42. Weber TR, Tracy TF Jr, Silen ML, et al. Enterostomy and its closure in newborns. Arch Surg 1995;130(5):534–7.
43. Voss M, Moore SW, van der Merwe I, et al. Fulminating necrotising enterocolitis: outcome and prognostic factors. Pediatr Surg Int 1998;13(8):576–80.
44. Ricketts RR, Jerles ML. Neonatal necrotizing enterocolitis: experience with 100 consecutive surgical patients. World J Surg 1990;14(5):600–5.
45. Ein SH, Marshall DG, Girvan D. Peritoneal drainage under local anesthesia for perforations from necrotizing enterocolitis. J Pediatr Surg 1977;12(6):963–7.
46. Lessin MS, Luks FI, Wesselhoeft CW Jr, et al. Peritoneal drainage as definitive treatment for intestinal perforation in infants with extremely low birth weight (<750 g). J Pediatr Surg 1998;33(2):370–2.
47. Morgan LJ, Shochat SJ, Hartman GE. Peritoneal drainage as primary management of perforated NEC in the very low birth weight infant. J Pediatr Surg 1994;29(2):310–4 [discussion: 314–5].
48. Gollin G, Abarbanell A, Baerg JE. Peritoneal drainage as definitive management of intestinal perforation in extremely low-birth-weight infants. J Pediatr Surg 2003; 38(12):1814–7.
49. Ein SH, Shandling B, Wesson D, et al. A 13-year experience with peritoneal drainage under local anesthesia for necrotizing enterocolitis perforation. J Pediatr Surg 1990;25(10):1034–6 [discussion: 1036–7].

50. Moss RL, Dimmitt RA, Barnhart DC, et al. Laparotomy versus peritoneal drainage for necrotizing enterocolitis and perforation. N Engl J Med 2006;354(21):2225–34.

51. Rees CM, Eaton S, Kiely EM, et al. Peritoneal drainage or laparotomy for neonatal bowel perforation? A randomized controlled trial. Ann Surg 2008;248(1):44–51.

52. Horwitz JR, Lally KP, Cheu HW, et al. Complications after surgical intervention for necrotizing enterocolitis: a multicenter review. J Pediatr Surg 1995;30(7):994–8 [discussion: 998–9].

53. Simon NP. Follow-up for infants with necrotizing enterocolitis. Clin Perinatol 1994; 21(2):411–24.

54. Janik JS, Ein SH, Mancer K. Intestinal stricture after necrotizing enterocolitis. J Pediatr Surg 1981;16(4):438–43.

55. Stringer MD, Brereton RJ, Drake DP, et al. Recurrent necrotizing enterocolitis. J Pediatr Surg 1993;28(8):979–81.

56. Ricketts RR. Surgical treatment of necrotizing enterocolitis and the short bowel syndrome. Clin Perinatol 1994;21(2):365–87.

57. Sondheimer JM, Sokol RJ, Narkewicz MR, et al. Anastomotic ulceration: a late complication of ileocolonic anastomosis. J Pediatr 1995;127(2):225–30.

58. Vohr BR, Wright LL, Dusick AM, et al. Neurodevelopmental and functional outcomes of extremely low birth weight infants in the National Institute of Child Health and Human Development Neonatal Research Network, 1993-1994. Pediatrics 2000;105(6):1216–26.

59. Sonntag J, Grimmer I, Scholz T, et al. Growth and neurodevelopmental outcome of very low birthweight infants with necrotizing enterocolitis. Acta Paediatr 2000; 89(5):528–32.

60. Hintz SR, Kendrick DE, Stoll BJ, et al. Neurodevelopmental and growth outcomes of extremely low birth weight infants after necrotizing enterocolitis. Pediatrics 2005;115(3):696–703.

61. Schulzke SM, Deshpande GC, Patole SK. Neurodevelopmental outcomes of very low-birth-weight infants with necrotizing enterocolitis: a systematic review of observational studies. Arch Pediatr Adolesc Med 2007;161(6):583–90.

62. Rees CM, Pierro A, Eaton S. Neurodevelopmental outcomes of neonates with medically and surgically treated necrotizing enterocolitis. Arch Dis Child Fetal Neonatal Ed 2007;92(3):F193–8.

63. Martin CR, Dammann O, Allred EN, et al. Neurodevelopment of extremely preterm infants who had necrotizing enterocolitis with or without late bacteremia. J Pediatr 2010;157(5):751–756.e1.

64. Blakely ML, Tyson JE, Lally KP, et al. Laparotomy versus peritoneal drainage for necrotizing enterocolitis or isolated intestinal perforation in extremely low birth weight infants: outcomes through 18 months adjusted age. Pediatrics 2006; 117(4):e680–7.

65. Pang KK, Chao NS, Wong BP, et al. The clip and drop back technique in the management of multifocal necrotizing enterocolitis: a single centre experience. Eur J Pediatr Surg 2012;22(1):85–90.

Biomarkers for Prediction and Diagnosis of Necrotizing Enterocolitis

Pak C. Ng, MD, FRCPCH*, Kathy Y.Y. Chan, PhD,
Terence C.W. Poon, PhD

KEYWORDS

- Biomarkers • Diagnosis • Necrotizing enterocolitis • Preterm • Infants

KEY POINTS

- Nonspecific biomarkers of the inflammatory cascade (eg, acute phase proteins, cytokines, and cell surface antigens) are unable to differentiate systemic infection from necrotizing enterocolitis (NEC).
- Gut-associated proteins may be used as specific biomarkers for bowel injury and for identifying critically ill patients with NEC who require surgical intervention.
- New molecular diagnostic techniques (eg, proteomics and microarrays) may in future assist neonatologists to discover unique biomarkers for specific organ injury or disease.

INTRODUCTION

Necrotizing enterocolitis (NEC) is a devastating gastrointestinal (GI) disease that predominantly affects preterm, very low birth weight (VLBW) infants. This condition is associated with high morbidity and mortality.[1,2] The estimated mortality rate ranges between 20% and 30%, and infants who require surgical intervention are at particularly high risk of dying from complications.[1] Classical NEC in preterm infants frequently presents in a fulminant manner with few antecedent signs but may progress rapidly to disseminated intravascular coagulation (DIC), multiorgan failure, and death within hours or days of clinical presentation.[3] In the acute phase, NEC infants may die from bowel perforation, pannecrosis of gut, peritonitis, and/or septicemia. In the chronic phase, NEC may also be associated with serious long-term complications, including short bowel syndrome, systemic infection, parenteral nutrition-associated

Conflict of Interest: Nil.
Financial Disclosure: Nil.
Department of Paediatrics, The Chinese University of Hong Kong, Shatin NT, Hong Kong SAR, The People's Republic of China
* Corresponding author. Department of Paediatrics, Prince of Wales Hospital, Level 6, Clinical Sciences Building, Shatin, New Territories, Hong Kong.
E-mail address: pakcheungng@cuhk.edu.hk

Clin Perinatol 40 (2013) 149–159
http://dx.doi.org/10.1016/j.clp.2012.12.005
0095-5108/13/$ – see front matter © 2013 Elsevier Inc. All rights reserved.

cholestasis, nutritional deficiency, and poor physical growth.[1] More importantly, it is now recognized that the intense immunoreactive response associated with bowel inflammation and necrosis can extend systemically to distant organs, in particular, the central nervous system, resulting in long-term neurodevelopmental impairments.[4,5] Thus, it is important to recognize the condition at the earliest time of onset so as to minimize bowel injury and limit the devastating effects of systemic immunoreactive response. However, early clinical manifestations of NEC are often nonspecific and may include common constitutional signs, such as unstable temperature, lethargy, poor peripheral perfusion, recurrent apnea, increase in oxygen, or ventilatory requirements, and vague abdominal signs, such as intolerance or regurgitation of milk and abdominal distension.[3] These signs and symptoms are rarely able to definitively differentiate NEC from other neonatal conditions such as exacerbation of bronchopulmonary dysplasia especially in infants on nasal continuous positive airway pressure with distended abdomen, GI dysmotility of prematurity, and electrolyte or sepsis-induced intestinal ileus.[3,6] In addition, early radiographic features of dilated bowel loops, thickened bowel walls, and paucity of intestinal gas in plain abdominal radiograph are difficult to interpret and have low sensitivity for diagnosing NEC.[7] Pneumatosis intestinalis, pneumoperitoneum, and portal venous gas are late signs and signify advanced disease. Other modalities of imaging such as Doppler ultrasonography, computed tomography, and magnetic resonance imaging scan of abdomen are either operator-dependent or require transport of sick preterm infants from the neonatal intensive care unit to the imaging room.

In the past 2 decades, several inflammatory mediators, such as acute phase proteins,[6,8–10] cytokines,[8,11] chemokines,[11] and cell surface antigens,[12–14] have been evaluated for early detection of NEC. More recently, advanced molecular and genetic techniques have further revolutionized the concept and approach in diagnostic medicine.[15] The objectives of this article are to examine emerging technologies and the potential usefulness of nonspecific and specific biomarkers for early diagnosis and identification of preterm infants at risk of developing NEC, as well as the use of such biomarkers in predicting the severity or outcome of the disease at the onset of clinical presentation.

PREDICTING INFANTS AT RISK OF DEVELOPING NEC

Clinical risk factors predisposed to NEC have long been recognized by neonatal clinicians. Although prematurity is considered to be the most important risk factor, other culprits including impaired perfusion of the GI tract such as absent or reverse end-diastolic flow in umbilical arteries,[16,17] patent ductus arteriosus, and exchange transfusion via umbilical vessels[18]; hypoxia such as cyanotic heart disease and low Apgar scores[18]; oxidative stress with reperfusion injury such as transfusion-related acute gut injury[19,20] and exposure to high oxygen concentration; and gut mucosal injury such as use of nonhuman milk formula and hypertonic feeds[18] have been incriminated in the etiology of NEC. Recently, much evidence suggests that the pathogenesis of NEC is mediated via complex interactions between genetic and environmental factors.[18] Hence, recognizing these adverse factors should be useful in early identification of preterm infants at increased risk of developing the condition.

Genetic Biomarkers

It is commonly observed that only a small subset of preterm infants develops NEC despite all infants in the cohort sharing a common environment and being treated in a standardized manner. This observation suggests that there may be inherited susceptibility to this condition and some infants are genetically programmed to be more vulnerable than others. The prime objectives of identifying genetic-environment interactions are (1) to understand the mechanism of disease, (2) to select susceptible patients who need close surveillance, and (3) to identify those who may benefit from targeted or personalized treatment.

In the past decade, much research has been focused on investigating whether inborn genetic differences can influence the likelihood of preterm infants developing NEC. The candidate-gene approach has been frequently adopted to assess the body immune mechanisms. In a retrospective cohort study, the -221 Y allele and mannose-binding lectin (MBL) 2 YY genotype were encountered significantly more frequently in infants with severe NEC than in control infants.[21] MBL is an important pattern recognition receptor of the innate immune system. The MBL2 genotypes could be associated with exaggerated inflammatory response and high circulating levels of MBL, contributing to intestinal damages.[22] In a prospective, multicenter cohort study of 271 VLBW infants, 15 had NEC, of whom 5 did not survive.[23] The investigators discovered that infants who developed NEC were significantly less mature and more likely to be of African-American origin. More importantly, they found that the *NFKB1* (g.24519 del ATTG) variant was present in all 15 infants with NEC but only in 65% of infants without NEC.[23] This genotype could reduce its target product binding to nuclear proteins, which would contribute to the impairment of mucosal immunity. Also, the *NFKB1A* (g.-1004A>G) variant was present in 13% and 49% of infants with and without NEC, respectively. The findings suggested that sequence variation in the toll-like receptor (TLR) pathway genes could select a subgroup of VLBW infants who would be at risk of developing the disease.[23] Another study indicated that the prevalence of IL-18[607] AA genotype was significantly more common in infants with stage III NEC compared with infants with stage I and II disease.[24] The genotype has been associated with increased IL-18 production, which could adversely affect the integrity of the intestinal barrier. In contrast, the prevalence of the mutant variant of IL-4 receptor α gene was higher in infants who did not develop the disease and implied that the presence of this variant gene might confer protection.[25] It was recognized that the variant gene could enhance the IL-4 signal transduction process and promote differentiation of lymphocyte into Th2 cells, which would be protective for the bowel mucosal barrier. In contrast, the IL-4 receptor α wild type allele, IL-4 receptor α AA, was associated with increased susceptibility to NEC. The presence of C allele in the gene encoding carbamoyl phosphate synthetase 1 (CPS1) (ie, CPS1 T1405N polymorphism) was also associated with increased risk of NEC.[26] It has been suggested that the decrease in L-arginine level could limit nitric oxide production, which would in turn disturb intestinal blood flow and interfere with the gut mucosal barrier integrity and function. Other investigators, however, failed to find any significant correlation between NEC and polymorphisms of other immune-related genes in various pathways connected to, for example, CD14, TLR-4, caspase-recruitment domain 15, and cytokines.[27,28]

The study of human genome and genetic polymorphisms are crucial for the future development of personalized medicine. However, major limitations of current genetic studies include (1) the lack of biologic functionality or explanation between the genetic findings and biochemical mechanisms, (2) an insufficient sample size, especially in rare conditions, to achieve adequate statistical power for validating outcomes, (3) a heterogenous group of patients, for example different ethnic and racial groups within the same cohort, and particularly in neonatology, different gestational and postnatal ages may also critically influence the results, and (4) the lack of homogeneity in the diagnosis. The latter issue is especially relevant to NEC because mild cases of NEC are often clinically and radiologically inconspicuous, and the diagnosis is often difficult to be confirmed by routine investigation. A positive association between a genetic biomarker and NEC would therefore require proper validation of its biologic functionality and confirmation by subsequent targeted clinical trials.[29] Despite its clinical importance, genetic polymorphisms have not been routinely used in preterm infants to assess the risk of NEC. Once the whole genome could be routinely screened at birth, it would be easier to evaluate gene interactions and the probability of preterm infants developing NEC.

Biomarkers of Oxidative Stress

Much evidence has accumulated in the past decade to suggest that oxidative stress and reperfusion injury may play a key role in the etiology of NEC. An impaired ability of preterm infants to neutralize free radicals and counteract products of oxidative stress can give rise to injury of gut epithelial cells and result in cellular necrosis and apoptosis. Consequently, this can manifest clinically as bowel inflammation or NEC. Thus, the determination of oxidative stress biomarkers at birth may theoretically allow identification of high-risk preterm infants who may benefit from close monitoring. In a multicenter study of 332 preterm newborns with gestational age ranging between 24 and 33 weeks, infants with NEC (n = 29) had significantly lower gestational age and birth weight and significantly higher cord blood levels of total hydroperoxides, advanced oxidation protein products, and nonprotein bound iron, compared with those without NEC (n = 303).[30] Although the results suggest an association between intrauterine oxidative stress and increase risk of NEC, further study is needed to determine the diagnostic usefulness (ie, sensitivity, specificity, predictive values, and accuracy) of these oxidative stress biomarkers as predictors of NEC.

Metagenomics

The microbial ecology of the GI tract has been documented to play a pivotal role in the development of bowel inflammation. The vast diversity of intestinal flora renders conventional culture and typing of bacteria redundant in the process of searching for evidence of their involvement in NEC. A recently developed technique is the use of metagenomics for molecular identification of a vast array of microorganisms. The high throughput 16S rRNA sequencing has been used for comprehensive analysis of gut microbiota and for identification of specific signatures of bacterial sequences in stool and tissue samples. A recent study demonstrated that a change in bacterial pattern in stool specimens with increase of *Proteobacteria* and decrease of *Firmicutes* could be associated with subsequent development of NEC in preterm infants.[31] Also, a case-control study of fecal specimens from 10 preterm infants with NEC and an equal number of matched control infants without NEC suggested that intestinal microbial colonization in NEC infants had low diversity of GI flora, with increase in abundance of *Proteobacteria* and decrease in other bacteria species.[32] Further, the bacterial composition and their relative number in inflamed bowel tissues surgically removed from NEC infants (n = 24) were determined by fluorescence *in situ* hybridization laser capture microdissection.[33] Although a significant correlation was observed between pneumatosis intestinalis and the presence of *C.butyicum/C. parputrificum*, a wide variation of microorganisms was present in the specimens and no dominating single pathogen or combination of pathogens was found. *Proteobacteria* (49.0%), *Firmicutes* (30.4%), *Actinobacteria* (17.1%), and *Bacteroidetes* (3.6%) were detected by 16S rRNA gene sequencing. Again, the relative dominance of *Proteobacteria* was observed and could explain the susceptibility of these preterm infants to NEC.[33] Further clinical evaluation is required to determine whether regular screening of stool microbiota could effectively predict the development of NEC in at-risk infants.[34]

EARLY DIAGNOSIS OF NEC

The breakdown of gut mucosal defense couples with overgrowth and invasion of micro-organisms through the GI tract may cause severe bowel damage and necrosis and induce marked systemic inflammatory responses. Currently used clinical biomarkers of NEC are usually pro or antiinflammatory mediators of the inflammatory cascade.[6,8–14] They include acute-phase proteins (eg, C-reactive protein [CRP], serum amyloid A [SAA], procalcitonin),[3,6,8–10] cytokines (eg, interleukin [IL] 6, IL-4, IL-10, tumor necrosis factor),[8,11] chemokines (eg, IL-8/CXC-motif ligand 8; interferon-γ-inducible protein [IP-10]/CXCL10; regulated on activation, normal T cell expressed and secreted [RANTES]/CC-motif ligand 5 [CCL5]),[11,35] and cell surface antigens (eg, neutrophil CD64 and CD11b).[3,12–14] All are "nonspecific" biomarkers that are efficient in detecting systemic inflammation but none can effectively differentiate between neonatal sepsis and NEC. In the past decade, more investigators have focused on studying "specific" biomarkers of NEC. Clinically, it is important to differentiate NEC from intestinal ileus secondary to neonatal sepsis, because the management differs substantially with regard to antibiotic coverage and the duration of enteral fasting and parenteral nutrition. Thus, the ideal biomarker for NEC should not be responsive to sepsis-induced inflammation but should react promptly and specifically to intestinal tissue injury. In addition, the magnitude of change of these biomarkers from baseline should be proportional to the degree of gut mucosal damage and thus, reflect the severity of intestinal tissue injury. The biomarkers should also be able to identify a subgroup of NEC infants at the onset of clinical presentation who subsequently require surgical intervention.

Nonspecific Biomarkers of NEC

Most of the biomarkers in this group are mediators of the inflammatory cascade. Although individual reports may suggest that some are superior than others,[10,36] most biomarkers have similar diagnostic properties. "Early warning" biomarkers such as IL-6,[8] IP-10/CXCL10,[11] neutrophil CD64,[3,12,13] and SAA[6,10] are promising in detecting neonatal sepsis, NEC, and systemic inflammation. However, these are unable to differentiate NEC from other inflammatory diseases or infection.[3,6,8,10–13] IL-6 level, the upstream regulator of CRP, increases in circulating concentration substantially soon after the initiation of the inflammatory cascade. Its serum level falls precipitously within 24 hours with appropriate treatment.[8] Similarly, neutrophil CD64 antigen increases expression promptly and conspicuously in the early phase of septi-cemia and NEC.[12,13] Neutrophil CD64 is considered as a sensitive (95%–97%) and specific (97%–99%) test for detecting systemic inflammation, and it has a distinct advantage over cytokines and chemokines that the increase in antigen expression can persist more than 24 hours after the initial insult, and therefore, allows a wider window of opportunity for obtaining a representative blood sample during normal working hours.[37] Nonetheless, the laboratory procedures for processing of specimens are expensive and labor intensive.[37] Two acute phase proteins are in common use clinically. CRP is classified as a "late warning" biomarker because its circulating level increases 6 to 8 hours after the initial triggering event.[8] CRP assay is cheap and is performed easily and routinely. Two important points worth noting are (1) the use of CRP can be combined with an "early warning" biomarker such as IL-6, IP-10, or neutrophil CD64 to enhance its diagnostic utilities by covering both the early (ie, within the first 6 hours) and late (ie, >6–48 hours) phases of infection/inflammation[8] and (2) serial CRP measurements are useful in monitoring the progress of disease.[9] A persistently elevated CRP level in infants with NEC usually signifies the development of complications[9] such as occult bowel perforation with continuing peritonitis, abdominal abscess formation, or the formation of an inflammatory abdominal mass with segments of necrotic bowel matted together. Another commonly used acute-phase protein is SAA.[6,10] The combined use of SAA and apolipoprotein CII as the ApoSAA score was effective in stratifying preterm infants with suspected sepsis/NEC into different risk categories.[6] The ApoSAA score allows frontline neonatologists to withhold antimicrobial treatment in 45% and early stoppage of antibiotics within 24 hours in another 16% of patients.[6] To the authors' knowledge, this has been the first report that identified all infected and NEC infants at the onset of clinical presentation and recommended neonatologists to confidently withhold antibiotic treatment in low-risk–suspected sepsis/NEC cases.[6]

Typically, the more severe the infection or bowel injury, the higher would be the inflammatory response and the magnitude of change in the levels of inflammatory mediators.[8,10,12,38] However, it would be difficult to stratify different levels of cutoff values for quantifying the severity of infection or NEC. The sequential use of anti and proinflammatory cytokines and chemokines, comprising IL-10, IL-6, and RANTES/CCL5, could be used as a prognostic model.[35] The algorithm using these biomarkers readily identified 100% of sepsis/NEC cases that subsequently developed DIC at the initial stage of clinical presentation.[35] Thus, the mediators could assist frontline neonatologists in identifying the most severely sick infants for intensive treatment and in targeting those with the highest risk of developing adverse outcomes.

In a recent study, the profiles of plasma immunoregulatory proteins between NEC and spontaneous intestinal perforation (SIP) infants were compared and potential novel mediators identified.[39] Significantly higher concentrations of angiopoietin 2, soluble type II IL-1 receptor, and soluble urokinase-type plasminogen activator receptor and significantly lower concentration of secreted form of receptor tyrosine-protein kinase ErbB3 were found in patients with NEC compared with SIP.[39] The study demonstrated plasmatic signatures of immunoregulatory proteins, and the magnitude of changes in these proteins were significantly more extensive in NEC infants, thus reflecting different pathophysiology and nature of gut injury between the 2 conditions.[39] These proteins should be further assessed in clinical trials to differentiate NEC from SIP or other more benign GI conditions, such as GI dysmotility of prematurity.

Other proteins such as anaphylatoxin (C5a),[36] procalcitonin,[10,40] e-selectin,[8,41] and platelet activating factor[42,43] have also been reported to be useful for early diagnosis of NEC, but most studies included small number of subjects and there was considerable heterogeneity in the study design.

Specific Biomarkers of NEC

The current direction of biomarker research has been focused on discovering organ and/or disease-specific biomarkers.[15] This approach is particularly relevant to NEC. Specific mediators that can indicate enterocyte injury or cell death are potentially useful. Fatty acid binding proteins (FABP), calprotectin, and other gut-related proteins such as claudin-3 have been evaluated for their effectiveness in diagnosing NEC and their abilities to identify severe cases that are at high risk of dying or requiring surgical intervention.[44–49]

In a nonischemic rodent model of NEC, intraluminal instillation of casein and acidified calcium gluconate have resulted in superficial villus blunting and necrosis.[50] The investigators also observed a rapid concomitant increase in serum intestinal-FABP (I-FABP) level from the baseline, but such changes were not detected with serum hexosaminidase in these animals.[50] In a follow-up human study, serum I-FABP was able to identify all cases (n = 7) of stage III NEC but only 3 of 24 infants with stage I or II disease.[45] Similar findings were also encountered in critically ill adult patients with abdominal sepsis.[51] Circulating I-FABP and liver FABP were significantly elevated in nonsurvivors than survivors, suggesting that there were more severe sepsis and hepatosplanchnic hypoperfusion–induced GI and hepatocellular damages in the former group of patients.[51] More recent studies have investigated these biomarkers in urinary specimens,[46,47] since the half-lives of these proteins are short in the bloodstream.[52] Although urinary I-FABP (>800 pg/mL) obtained within the first 90 hours of life could predict all infants (n = 9) who subsequently developed stage II or III disease, the overall diagnostic utilities were not favourable as there were much overlap of urinary I-FABP levels among the non-NEC, stage I NEC, and stage II/III NEC groups.[46] Longitudinal monitoring of urinary I-FABP levels also failed to demonstrate its usefulness as a biomarker for predicting or screening of NEC before the onset clinical manifestations.[47] However, urinary I-FABP/creatinine ratio (>2.20 pg/nmol creatinine), urinary claudin-3 (>800.8 INT), and fecal calprotectin (>286.2 μg/g feces) were found to be promising for diagnosing NEC in the acute phase.[47] In particular, urinary I-FABP/creatinine ratio has sensitivity and specificity of 93% and 90% for differentiating NEC from non-NEC cases. A higher cut-off ratio at 6.38 pg/nmol creatinine could further identify infants who required surgery and nonsurvivors (sensitivity and specificity of 100% and 86%), suggesting that this urinary biomarker has the capability to select the most critically ill cases and could guide the decision for surgical exploration.[47] In addition, urinary claudin-3 and fecal calprotectin have sensitivity of 71% and 86% and specificity of 81% and 93%, respectively. The latter 2 biomarkers were, however, not correlated with the disease severity.[47] Another study that monitored fecal calprotectin level longitudinally also suggested that it was useful for identifying established NEC cases and severe GI inflammatory conditions but could not be used for screening as the increase in fecal calprotectin level could not predate the occurrence of abdominal signs and symptoms.[49] The main disadvantage of using urinary and fecal samples was that a time-dependent collection such as a 24-hour urine sample would be notoriously difficult to collect especially in female subjects, infants under radiant heater, and sick patients with rapidly deteriorating renal function, as well as fecal samples in infants with intestinal ileus after the development of NEC. Further multicenter studies should be conducted to fully delineate the effectiveness and limitations of using these gut-specific biomarkers for diagnosis of the condition.

A potentially new class of GI diagnostic biomarker is microRNA (miRNA). miRNAs are small noncoding RNA segments (~22 nucleotides) that may inhibit gene expression for producing functional proteins. This class of nucleic acids has been used as diagnostic biomarkers for detecting sepsis in adults[53] and differentiating different types of bowel inflammation (eg, Crohn disease vs ulcerative colitis) in different locations (eg, terminal ileum vs colon) of the GI tract.[54] Theoretically, similar techniques and principles may apply to NEC, thereby allowing frontline neonatal clinicians and surgeons to promptly diagnose the condition and more importantly, to locate the exact sites of diseased bowel for surgery.

SEARCHING FOR "NOVEL" BIOMARKERS OF NEC

The prime objective of biomarker research is the identification of novel and previously unreported biomarkers for clinical applications.[6,15] Advances in molecular diagnostic techniques especially in nucleic acid sequencing and mass screening methods, such as proteomics and microarray technologies, have revolutionized the approach for discovering new biomarkers.[15] In brief, the principle consists of 2 distinctive phases: the biomarker discovery phase and the independent validation phase.[6] Firstly, in the biomarker discovery phase, a case-control comparsion of mediator profiles such as plasma protein profiles from proteomics study or nucleic acids profiles from sequencing between NEC and control subjects can be used for selecting the desired mediators. The selected mediators will only be considered as potential biomarkers if they can demonstrate a reversal pattern of response upon disease recovery or with appropriate treatment in a subsequent longitudinal study conducted in a separate group of patients. This important step is essential to exclude mediators due to systematic bias. Secondly, in the validation phase, the selected mediators will then be subjected to further evaluation by a prospective cohort study to determine the diagnostic utilities, including sensitivity, specificity, positive, and negative predictive values, and accuracy of these mediators.[6] Recently, the authors' research team has stringently followed this protocol and successfully used the mass spectrometry-based proteomic profiling technique to identify known and novel host-response signature proteins, SAA, and proapolipoprotein CII for early diagnosis of neonatal sepsis and NEC.[6] Thus, new technologies couple with stringent study design would enable the discovery of novel and robust biomarkers for specific organ injury or a disease entity.

THE FUTURE

Recent advances in sophisticated molecular and genetic diagnostic technologies have greatly opened up new opportunities in biomarker research. The development of next-generation sequencing (NGS) has considerably improved the sensitivity and resolution, as well as efficiency in terms of high throughput, scalability, and speed of nucleic acids sequencing in plasma and tissues.[55] Obviously, diseases with known genetic defects such as Down syndrome and other trisomy fetuses could be targeted for noninvasive antenatal screening. In recent studies, Down fetuses were detected with extremely high accuracy by demonstrating the presence of minute but significantly increased quantity of chromosome 21 sequences in maternal blood.[56,57] Such breakthrough in diagnostic technology would undoubtedly revolutionize future concepts of biomarker discovery and disease screening. Theoretically, NGS can be applied for detecting specific nucleic acids, in particular, mRNA, miRNA, and methylated DNA in different biologic tissues, and allows accurate screening and/or diagnosis of gut inflammation and necrosis. Other powerful mass screening techniques such as microarrays and proteomics will also permit different types of molecules to be studied. In future, neonatal clinicians will use these emerging new technologies to actively search for new and specific biomarkers for diagnosing and assessing the severity of NEC.

SUMMARY

This review has summarized the commonly used biomarkers currently available for diagnosis of necrotizing enterocolitis. The most exciting advances in diagnostic tests were the use of new nucleic acid sequencing techniques (eg, next-generation sequencing) and molecular screening methods (eg, proteomics and microarray analysis) for the discovery of novel biomarkers. The new technology platform coupled with stringent protocols of biomarker discovery and validation would enable neonatologists to study biologic systems at a level never before possible and discover unique biomarkers for specific organ injury and/or disease entity.[6,15]

REFERENCES

1. Neu J, Walker WA. Necrotizing enterocolitis. N Engl J Med 2011;364(3):255–64.
2. Lin PW, Stoll BJ. Necrotising enterocolitis. Lancet 2006;368(10):1271–83.

3. Lam HS, Wong SP, Cheung HM, et al. Early diagnosis of intra-abdominal inflammation and sepsis by neutrophil CD64 expression in newborns. Neonatology 2011;99(2):118–24.
4. Hintz SR, Kendrick DE, Stoll BJ, et al. Neurodevelopmental and growth outcomes of extremely low birth weight infants after necrotizing enterocolitis. Pediatrics 2005;115(3):696–703.
5. Salhab WA, Perlman JM, Silver L, et al. Necrotizing enterocolitis and neurodevelopmental outcome in extremely low birth weight infants <1000 g. J Perinatol 2004; 24(9):534–40.
6. Ng PC, Ang IL, Chiu RW, et al. Host-response biomarkers for diagnosis of late-onset septicemia and necrotizing enterocolitis in preterm infants. J Clin Invest 2010;120(8):2989–3000.
7. Kosloske AM, Musemeche CA, Ball WS Jr, et al. Necrotizing enterocolitis: value of radiographic findings to predict outcome. Am J Roentgenol 1988;151(4): 771–4.
8. Ng PC, Cheng SH, Chui KM, et al. Diagnosis of late onset neonatal sepsis with cytokines, adhesion molecule, and C-reactive protein in preterm very low birth weight infants. Arch Dis Child Fetal Neonatal Ed 1997;77(3):221–7.
9. Pourcyrous M, Korones SB, Yang W, et al. C-reactive protein in the diagnosis, management and prognosis of neonatal necrotizing enterocolitis. Pediatrics 2005;116(5):1064–9.
10. Centinkaya M, Ozkan H, Koksal N, et al. Comparison of the efficacy of serum amyloid A, C-reactive protein, and procalcitonin in the diagnosis and follow-up of necrotizing enterocolitis in premature infants. J Pediatr Surg 2011;46(8): 1482–9.
11. Ng PC, Li K, Chui KM, et al. IP-10 is an early diagnostic marker for identification of late-onset bacterial infection in preterm infants. Pediatr Res 2007;61(1):93–8.
12. Ng PC, Li K, Wong RP, et al. Neutrophil CD64 expression: a sensitive diagnostic marker for late-onset nosocomial infection in very low birth weight infants. Pediatr Res 2002;51(3):296–303.
13. Bhandari V, Wang C, Rinder C, et al. Hematologic profile of sepsis in neonates: neutrophil CD64 as a diagnostic marker. Pediatrics 2008;121(1):129–34.
14. Turunen R, Andersson S, Nupponen I, et al. Increased CD11b-density on circulating phagocytes as an early sign of late-onset sepsis in extremely low-birth-weight infants. Pediatr Res 2005;57(2):270–5.
15. Ng PC, Lam HS. Biomarkers in neonatology: the next generation of test. Neonatology 2012;102(2):145–51.
16. Kirsten GF, van Zyl N, Smith M, et al. Necrotizing enterocolitis in infants born to women with severe early preeclampsia and absent end-diastolic umbilical artery Doppler flow velocity waveforms. Am J Perinatol 1999;16(6):309–14.
17. Kamoji VM, Dorling JS, Manktelow B, et al. Antenatal umbilical Doppler abnormalities: an independent risk factor for early onset neonatal necrotizing enterocolitis in premature infants. Acta Paediatr 2008;97(3):327–31.
18. Young C, Sharma R, Handfield M, et al. Biomarkers for infants at risk for necrotizing enterocolitis: clues to prevention? Pediatr Res 2009;65(5):91R–7R.
19. Blau J, Calo JM, Dozor D, et al. Transfusion-related acute gut injury: necrotizing enterocolitis in very low birth weight neonates after packed red blood cell transfusion. J Pediatr 2011;158(3):403–9.
20. Singh R, Visintainer PF, Frantz ID, et al. Association of necrotizing enterocolitis with anemia and packed red blood cell transfusions in preterm infants. J Perinatol 2011; 31(1):176–82.

21. Prencipe G, Azzari C, Moriondo M, et al. Association between mannose-binding lectin gene polymorphisms and necrotizing enterocolitis in preterm infants. J Pediatr Gastroenterol Nutr 2012;55(2):160–5.

22. IP WK, Takahashi K, Ezekowitz RA, et al. Mannose-binding lectin and innate immunity. Immunol Rev 2009;230(1):9–21.

23. Sampath V, Le M, Lane L, et al. The NFKB1 (g.-24519delATTG) variant is associated with necrotizing enterocolitis (NEC) in premature infants. J Surg Res 2011; 169(1):e51–7.

24. Heninger E, Treszl A, Kocsis I, et al. Genetic varients of the interleukin-18 promoter region (-607) influence the course of necrotizing enterocolitis in very low birth weight neonates. Eur J Pediatr 2002;161(7):410–1.

25. Treszl A, Heninger A, Kalman A, et al. Low prevalence of IL-4 receptor alpha-chain gene G variant in very-low-birth-weight infants with necrotizing enterocolitis. J Pediatr Surg 2003;38(9):1374–8.

26. Moonen RM, Paulussen AD, Souren NY, et al. Carbamoyl phosphate synthetase polymorphisms as a risk factor for necrotizing enterocolitis. Pediatr Res 2007; 62(2):188–90.

27. Szebeni B, Szekeres R, Rusai K, et al. Genetic polymorphisms of CD14, toll-like receptor 4, and caspase-recruitment domain 15 are not associated with necrotizing enterocolitis in very low birth weight infants. J Pediatr Gastroenterol Nutr 2006;42(1):27–31.

28. Henderson G, Craig S, Baier RJ, et al. Cytokine gene polymorphisms in preterm infants with necrotising enterocolitis: genetic association study. Arch Dis Child Fetal Neonatal Ed 2009;94(2):F124–8.

29. Harding D. Impact of common genetic variation on neonatal disease and outcome. Arch Dis Child Fetal Neonatal Ed 2007;92(5):F408–13.

30. Perrone S, Tataranno ML, Negro S, et al. May oxidative stress biomarkers in cord blood predict the occurrence of necrotizing enterocolitis in preterm infants? J Matern Fetal Neonatal Med 2012;25(Suppl 1):128–31.

31. Mai V, Young CM, Ukhanova M, et al. Fecal microbiota in premature infants prior to necrotizing enterocolitis. PLoS One 2011;6:e20647.

32. Wang Y, Hoenig JD, Malin KJ, et al. 16S rRNA gene-based analysis of fecal microbiota from preterm infants with and without necrotizing enterocolitis. ISME J 2009;3(8):944–54.

33. Smith B, Bode S, Petersen BL, et al. Community analysis of bacteria colonizing intestinal tissue of neonates with necrotizing enterocolitis. BMC Microbiol 2011;11(4):73.

34. Morowitz MJ, Denef VJ, Costello EK, et al. Strain-resolved community genomic analysis of gut microbial colonization in a premature infants. Proc Natl Acad Sci U S A 2011;108(3):1128–33.

35. Ng PC, Li K, Leung TF, et al. Early prediction of sepsis-induced disseminated intravascular coagulation with interleukin-10, interleukin-6, and RANTES in preterm infants. Clin Chem 2006;52(6):1181–9.

36. Tayman C, Tonbul A, Kahveci H, et al. C5a, a complement activation product, is a useful marker in predicting the severity of necrotizing enterocolitis. Tohoku J Exp Med 2011;224(2):143–50.

37. Ng PC, Lam HS. Biomarkers for late-onset neonatal sepsis: cytokines and beyond. Clin Perinatol 2010;37(3):599–610.

38. Ng PC, Li K, Wong RP, et al. Proinflammatory and anti-inflammatory cytokine responses in preterm infants with systemic infections. Arch Dis Child Fetal Neonatal Ed 2003;88(3):209–13.

39. Chan KY, Leung FW, Lam HS, et al. Immunoregulatory protein profiles of necro-tizing enterocolitis *versus* spontaneous intestinal perforation in preterm infants. PLoS One 2012;7(5):e36977.
40. Turner D, Hammerman C, Rudensky B, et al. Low levels of procalcitonin during episodes of necrotizing enterocolitis. Dig Dis Sci 2007;52(11):2972–6.
41. Khoo AK, Hall NJ, Alexander N, et al. Plasma soluble e-selectin in necrotizing enterocolitis. Eur J Pediatr Surg 2008;18(6):419–22.
42. Kultursay N, Kantar M, Akisu M, et al. Platelet-activating factor concentrations in healthy and septic neonates. Eur J Pediatr 1999;158(9):740–1.
43. Caplan MS, Sun XM, Hseuh W, et al. Role of platelet activating factor and tumor necrosis factor-alpha in neonatal necrotizing enterocolitis. J Pediatr 1990;116(6): 960–4.
44. Aydemir C, Dilli D, Oguz SS, et al. Serum intestinal fatty acid binding protein level for early diagnosis and prediction of severity of necrotizing enterocolitis. Early Hum Dev 2011;87(10):659–61.
45. Edelson MB, Sonnino RE, Bagwell CE, et al. Plasma intestinal fatty acid binding protein in neonates with necrotizing enterocolitis: a pilot study. J Pediatr Surg 1999;34(10):1453–7.
46. Mannoia K, Boskovic DS, Slater L, et al. Necrotizing enterocolitis is associated with neonatal intestinal injury. J Pediatr Surg 2011;46(1):81–5.
47. Thuijls G, Derikx JP, van Wijck K, et al. Non-invasive markers for early diagnosis and determination of the severity of necrotizing enterocolitis. Ann Surg 2010; 251(6):1174–80.
48. Campeotto F, Baldassarre M, Butel MJ, et al. Fecal calprotectin: cutoff values for identifying intestinal distress in preterm infants. J Pediatr Gastroenterol Nutr 2009;48(4):507–10.
49. Josefsson S, Bunn SK, Domellof M. Fecal calprotectin in very low birth weight infants. J Pediatr Gastroenterol Nutr 2007;44(4):407–13.
50. Gollin G, Marks WH. Elevation of circulating intestinal fatty acid binding protein in a luminal contents – Initiated model of NEC. J Pediatr Surg 1993;28(3):367–71.
51. Derikx JP, Poeze M, van Bijnen AA, et al. Evidence for intestinal and liver epithelial cell injury in the early phase of sepsis. Shock 2007;28(5):544–8.
52. van de Poll MC, Derikx JP, Buurman WA, et al. Liver manipulation causes hepa-tocyte injury and precedes system inflammation in patients undergoing liver resection. World J Surg 2007;31(10):2033–8.
53. Vasilescu C, Rossi S, Shimizu M, et al. MicroRNA fingerprints identify miR-150 as a plasma prognostic marker in patients with sepsis. PLoS One 2009;4:e7405.
54. Wu F, Zhang S, Dassopoulos T, et al. Identification of microRNAs associated with ileal and colonic Crohn's disease. Inflamm Bowel Dis 2010;16(10):1729–38.
55. Voelkerding KV, Dames SA, Durtschi JD. Next-generation sequencing: from basic research to diagnostics. Clin Chem 2009;54(4):641–58.
56. Chiu RW, Cantor CR, Lo YM. Non-invasive prenatal diagnosis by single molecule counting technologies. Trends Genet 2009;25(7):324–31.
57. Chiu RW, Akolekar R, Zheng YW, et al. Non-invasive prenatal assessment of trisomy 21 by multiplexed maternal plasma DNA sequencing: large scale validity study. BMJ 2011;342:c7401.

Intestinal Transplantation in Infants with Intestinal Failure

Richard S. Mangus, MD, MS[a],*, Girish C. Subbarao, MD[b]

KEYWORDS

- Intestinal failure • Intestinal rehabilitation • Intestinal transplantation
- Necrotizing enterocolitis • Parenteral nutrition

KEY POINTS

- Intestinal failure results from the inability of functional intestine to provide adequate nutrition and hydration to maintain growth and development and to support life.
- Intestinal rehabilitation includes a combination of medical and surgical management techniques implemented in patients with intestinal failure to return enteral autonomy.
- Intestinal transplantation is available to those children with intestinal failure who are not candidates for, or who fail, intestinal rehabilitation.
- Timing of referral for intestinal transplantation affects long-term survival; patients with late referral carry a higher risk of mortality, or may require complex multiorgan transplantation.
- Outcomes for intestinal transplantation show good patient growth and development, quality of life, and relative cost-effectiveness; there are inadequate data for the long-term durability of the intestinal graft.

INTRODUCTION

Necrotizing enterocolitis (NEC) is one of several intestinal disorders of infancy that can lead to intestinal dysfunction. Examples of other surgical diseases affecting the abdominal gastrointestinal tract include duodenal atresia or web; atresia of the jejunum, ileum, or large intestine; and volvulus. These disease states are generally related to organ blood flow, including either inadequate flow from hypotension or excess intestinal demand, or an in utero vascular accident preventing normal development. These disorders frequently require surgical intervention with resection resulting in a state historically known as short-gut syndrome. However, other disease processes of the intestine exist, with normal intestinal length, and these may also result in intestinal dysfunction. Patients with gastroschisis, Hirschsprung disease, intestinal malrotation, microvillus inclusion disease, and tufting enteropathy may have full intestinal length but

[a] Transplant Division, Department of Surgery, Indiana University School of Medicine, 550 North University Boulevard, Room 4601, Indianapolis, IN 46202-5250, USA; [b] Department of Pediatrics, Indiana University School of Medicine, 705 Riley Hospital Drive, ROC 4210, Indianapolis, IN 46202, USA
* Corresponding author.
E-mail address: rmangus@iupui.edu

Clin Perinatol 40 (2013) 161–173
http://dx.doi.org/10.1016/j.clp.2012.12.010
0095-5108/13/$ – see front matter © 2013 Elsevier Inc. All rights reserved.
perinatology.theclinics.com

inadequate function. Intestinal failure (IF) is now defined as the inability of the functional intestinal mass to provide adequate nutrition and hydration to maintain normal growth and development, and to support life. IF can occur exclusive of intestinal length.[1,2]

Management of IF has evolved significantly in the last decade, with a greater number of successful therapeutic options and decreased patient morbidity and mortality.[3] However, as with any rapidly advancing field, controversy now exists regarding the appropriate use and timing of each of these interventions to optimize patient outcomes. The mainstay of therapy for IF is intravenous parenteral nutrition (PN). PN directly replaces both the nutrition and hydration required for growth and development and to sustain life. However, long-term PN is fraught with life-threatening complications including recurrent blood stream infections and sepsis, and venous thrombosis and sclerosis, which result in loss of vascular access, chronic electrolyte abnormalities, and dehydration, which can result in renal failure, and liver cirrhosis, which can result in end-stage liver disease. Intestinal rehabilitation has evolved as a defined subspecialty, specifically targeting patients with IF with the goal of returning those patients to enteral autonomy to avoid the complications of long-term PN. Intestinal rehabilitation combines innovative medical and surgical therapies to accomplish this goal.

However, certain patients are not candidates for intestinal rehabilitation or fail this management approach.[4,5] These patients may be candidates for intestinal transplantation (IT). IT is now the standard of care for patients with IF who fail standard medical and surgical options. Patients with very short intestinal length, full-length Hirschsprung, or functional enteropathies may never tolerate enteral feedings and should be referred immediately for intestinal transplantation, before they develop the complications associated with PN. Other patients may spend months and years undergoing medical and surgical interventions, but never achieve enteral autonomy.[6,7] As they begin to develop complications of PN, they should be referred for evaluation for IT.[8,9] Criteria for referral and for listing for IT are listed in **Table 1**.[3] Risk factors in

Table 1
Recommended criteria for consultation or referral for intestinal transplant assessment and for transplant listing

Referral Criteria	Listing Criteria
Children with massive intestine resection	Small intestine length of <25 cm without an ileocecal valve
Children with severely diseased intestine and unacceptable morbidity	IF with high morbidity and poor quality of life
Microvillus inclusion disease or intestinal epithelial dysplasia	Congenital intractable mucosal disorder such as microvillus inclusion disease or tufting enteropathy
Persistent hyperbilirubinemia (>6 mg/dL)	Persistent hyperbilirubinemia (>3–6 mg/dL) and signs of portal hypertension or synthetic liver dysfunction with coagulopathy
Thrombosis of 2 of 4 upper body central veins (jugular and subclavian)	Loss of more than 50% of the standard central venous access sites
Continuing prognostic or diagnostic uncertainty	Recurrent life-threatening episodes of sepsis resulting in multiorgan failure, metastatic infectious foci, or acquisition of flora with limited sensitivities
Request of patient or family	—

Adapted from Avitzur Y, Grant D. Intestine transplantation in children: update 2010. Pediatr Clin North Am 2010;57:418; with permission.

children with IF that may indicate referral to an intestinal rehabilitation center are listed in **Box 1.**[7]

The basis for referral for IT has changed significantly in the last decade. The development of new PN therapies that delay or reverse IF-associated liver disease (IFALD) has prolonged the time available to clinicians to reach enteral autonomy.[10–12] Use of ethanol and antibiotic locks for central venous catheters has decreased the rates of blood stream infections.[13] Intestinal lengthening procedures have increased in volume and improved in success.[14] These advances improve early patient outcomes, and delay the onset of PN-associated complications.[15] At this time, it is unclear whether they affect the overall long-term outcomes for high-risk patients. The controversy over timing for referral is ongoing and changes with advances in IF patient management and improved IT outcomes and quality of life (QOL).

Since the inception of IT, there have been more than 2000 of these procedures worldwide.[3] A large percentage of these patients are followed in the Intestinal Transplant Registry, with results reported every other year at the meetings of the Intestinal Transplant Association. More than one-half of these transplants were performed at one of 3 US centers: University of Pittsburgh, University of Nebraska, and University of Miami, although volumes at these centers have decreased in recent years. For the last 4 years, the largest center by volume has been Indiana University. There remain a limited number of IT centers worldwide with adequate volume to maintain proficiency. There is a steep learning curve associated with IT, as well as substantial costs associated with initiating a program. For this reason, most children in need of evaluation for IT must be referred to one of the active regional centers for care.

THERAPEUTIC OPTIONS AND/OR SURGICAL TECHNIQUE

Clinical care for children with IF is best provided by a multidisciplinary team including pediatricians, pediatric surgeons, transplant surgeons, nurses, dieticians, pharmacists, social workers, speech pathologists, and developmental specialists. There are

---

Box 1
Risk factors in children with IF that may indicate referral to an intestinal rehabilitation center

Pediatric risk factors prompting referral to an intestinal rehabilitation/transplant center

Prematurity and young age; less than 2 years of age

Poor mucosal integrity, ischemia (primary mucosal disorder)

Lack of ileocecal valve and residual small intestine length (<25 cm)

Intractable diarrhea

Early catheter infections (before 3 months of age)

More than 3 catheter infections or more than 1 infection per month

Excess lipid infusion (>3.5 g/kg/d)

Hyperbilirubinemia, thrombocytopenia, ascites, splenomegaly

Lack of enteral feeding

Lack of specialist staff; continuing prognostic or diagnostic uncertainty

Adapted from Beath S, Pironi L, Gabe S, et al. Collaborative strategies to reduce mortality and morbidity in patients with chronic intestinal failure including those who are referred for small bowel transplantation. Transplantation 2008;5:1381; with permission.

several novel therapeutic interventions that have evolved in recent years with demonstrated effectiveness. The use of intestinal lengthening procedures can achieve greater or full enteral autonomy. Lipid minimization formulations and protocols have been shown to minimize or reverse the progression of liver fibrosis. Gut trophic factors may help in maintaining mucosal integrity to prevent bacterial translocation from the intestinal lumen to the blood stream. Empiric antibiotic therapy may similarly be used to prevent bacterial overgrowth. The meticulous care of central venous catheters, along with ethanol and antibiotic locks, have been shown to lower the rates of catheter infections. In addition, the use of intestinal transplantation has shown improved clinical outcomes, although long-term data remain sparse. The remainder of this article focuses on intestinal transplantation.

Intestinal transplantation in children is limited to 3 primary procedures[1]: isolated transplantation of the small intestine (with or without the portion of the right colon with the ileocecal valve),[2] combined transplantation of the intestine and liver as separate grafts, and[3] multivisceral transplantation (MVT), which is the simultaneous transplantation of a composite graft including the liver, stomach, duodenum, pancreas, and small intestine (with or without the portion of the right colon with the ileocecal valve). Choice of transplant graft is made on a case-by-case basis depending on the patient's anatomy, disease process, previous surgeries, and immunologic makeup. The intestine and multivisceral transplants are shown in **Figs. 1** and **2**.

Transplantation of the small intestine as an isolated graft assumes normal function of the other organs of the abdomen. Pretransplantation evaluation of the abdominal organs includes upper gastrointestinal imaging (to assess the anatomy of the stomach and duodenum), gastric emptying evaluation, liver biopsy (to assess for fibrosis), and biopsy of the large intestine (to assess for ganglia). Kidney function is also assessed

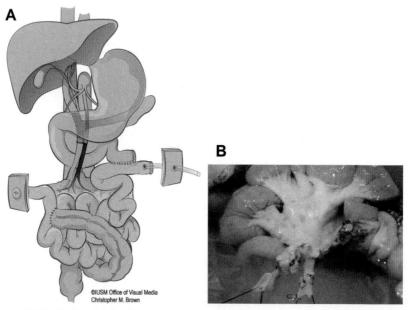

Fig. 1. (*A*) The isolated intestine transplant graft with arterial inflow from the superior mesenteric artery and venous outflow through the superior mesenteric vein (to the portal vein). (*B*) Isolated intestine graft showing superior mesenteric artery and vein. ([A] *Courtesy of* Indiana University School of Medicine, Indianapolis, IN; with permission.)

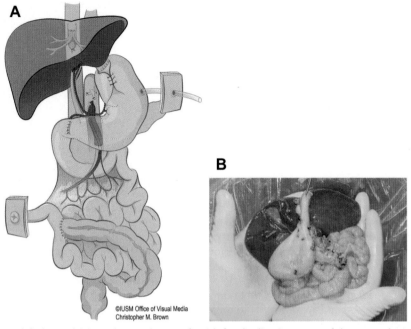

Fig. 2. (*A*) The multivisceral transplant graft with fundoplication wrap of the stomach. Arterial inflow is from the aorta to a common cuff of the celiac trunk and the superior mesenteric artery, with venous outflow through the portal system, into the liver, and through the hepatic veins into the vena cava. (*B*) The pediatric multivisceral composite graft including liver, stomach, duodenum, pancreas, and small intestine. ([A] *Courtesy of* Indiana University School of Medicine, Indianapolis, IN; with permission.)

because simultaneous kidney transplantation is possible. The vasculature is assessed for patency by computed tomography scan with arterial and venous phases. The transplant graft derives inflow through the superior mesenteric artery and outflow through the superior mesenteric vein. The recipient inflow can be provided by direct anastomosis to the native superior mesenteric artery or to the abdominal aorta inferior to the renal arteries. Outflow can be directed through the native superior mesenteric vein to the portal vein with flow through the liver. If this outflow path is inadequate, the donor superior mesenteric vein can be anastomosed directly to the recipient vena cava inferior to the renal veins. This outflow tract bypasses the liver, thereby necessitating hepatic metabolism of absorbed nutrients through a second-pass effect. Enteric anastomoses are formed between the recipient and donor proximal jejunum and between the recipient large intestine and the donor terminal ileum. This lower anastomosis is formed 10 to 15 cm from the end of the terminal ileum in a chimney fashion; this end segment is then passed through the abdominal wall as a terminal ileostomy. The ileostomy serves to decompress the intestine to avoid undue tension on the new anastomosis and also offers ready access for endoscopy for surveillance and biopsy of the intestinal graft.

Multivisceral transplantation is more technically demanding than transplantation of the intestine alone. Combined transplantation of the liver and small intestine comprises an isolated liver transplant and an isolated small intestine transplant. However, a full multivisceral transplant includes complete resection of the recipient liver, stomach, duodenum, pancreas, small intestine, and a portion of the large intestine. The resection alone is a significant undertaking, leaving the patient with an abdomen devoid of organs, except the kidneys and bladder. The donor graft derives vascular inflow from a combined patch of the celiac trunk and the superior mesenteric artery. The blood perfuses all of the transplant organs, with outflow through the superior mesenteric vein and splenic vein, which join to form the portal vein with flow into the liver. The outflow from the liver is through the 3 hepatic veins, which are sewn to the recipient hepatic veins. Therefore, there is a single arterial inflow from the native aorta to a patch of the donor celiac trunk and the superior mesenteric artery, with venous outflow through the hepatic veins into the recipient vena cava and right atrium. Enteric anastomoses are formed between the recipient and donor stomachs or the recipient esophagus and donor stomach. The transplant stomach is transplanted in its entirety because it experiences improved peristalsis and emptying as a whole organ. The recipient large intestine and the donor terminal ileum are connected as previously described with a terminal ileostomy.

Reperfusion of the graft results in immediate blood flow throughout the transplanted organs. Intestinal peristalsis can generally be seen within 60 seconds of reperfusion and often the small intestine experiences a hyperperistaltic period for several minutes after reperfusion. For the multivisceral graft, there is also immediate function of the pancreas (blood glucose control) and liver (production of bile, glucose, and blood clotting factors). At some centers, enteral feedings begin immediately, whereas others use only a dextrose drip for several days before starting elemental enteral feedings. As the enteral feedings are increased, posttransplant PN is decreased at a corresponding rate. Complete weaning from PN to enteral nutrition in an uncomplicated transplant usually occurs within 2 to 3 weeks of transplantation. For patients with hyperbilirubinemia, the bilirubin levels start to normalize as the PN is lowered and then stopped. Depending on the amount of liver injury experienced, bilirubin levels can return to normal within 4 to 8 weeks of stopping PN.

Choice of the donor graft depends on size and blood type, as well as donor quality. Donors as young as 7 weeks of age have been successfully used for multivisceral transplantation at our center. The median wait time for isolated intestine transplant in the United States is 6 to 8 months, but varies greatly depending on the individual transplant center. The transplant wait time for patients with advanced liver fibrosis or cirrhosis awaiting a multiorgan graft can be significantly longer because the patient moves into the pool of all patients awaiting a liver transplant, which not only increases wait-list time but increases mortality risk significantly. This difference in wait-list time and mortality risk underscores the importance of timely referral for intestinal transplantation. If patients can avoid significant liver damage from PN, and they ultimately fail intestinal rehabilitation, they remain a candidate for isolated small intestine transplant with its short wait-list time and lesser mortality risk.

The loss of abdominal domain in patients with an extensive surgical history results in closure of the abdominal wall being a particular challenge.[16] Various approaches to accomplishing this task have been described. First, when given the option, a donor should be 50% to 75% of the size of the recipient. The proportionally smaller organs facilitate closure of the abdominal wall. Second, graft reduction can be used to cut down the transplanted large or small intestine, or liver, to provide additional space for closure. Nonfunctional kidneys can be resected. Third, component separation techniques have been described in which the component muscle layers of the abdominal wall are incised and separated to lengthen the reach of the edges. Fourth, both biological and synthetic implants have been described. The most complex implant is transplantation of the donor abdominal wall, which implants the anterior abdominal wall (skin, subcutaneous tissue, muscle/fascia layers, and peritoneum) on a pedicle of the inferior epigastric artery and vein (**Fig. 3**). If sufficient native skin is present for

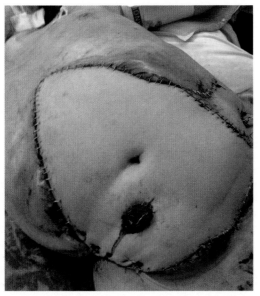

Fig. 3. Abdominal wall transplant in a teenager following multivisceral transplantation.

coverage of the fascia, a mesh can be implanted to reconstruct the fascia layer of the abdomen. Skin flaps can then be raised and brought together to cover the mesh implant. Biological meshes that are commonly used come from human fascia, human dermis, and pig dermis.[17,18] Synthetic meshes are less commonly used because of risk of infection and an association with enterocutaneous fistula formation caused by erosion of the mesh into the friable small intestine graft (**Fig. 4**A, B).

CLINICAL OUTCOMES

Of all intestinal transplantations, approximately 50% occur in adult patients, leaving 50% in the pediatric population.[3] Most surviving patients are able to live at home, taking an oral diet, and are free from PN. Overall, short-term survival has improved

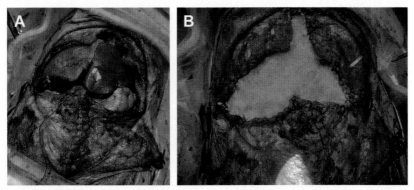

Fig. 4. (*A*) A complex closure of the abdominal wall, with remaining large fascial defect after partial closure of the inferior fascia. A portion of the right lobe of the liver has been resected to provide additional space. (*B*) The previous abdominal wall with acellular dermal allograft (human) placed to reconstruct the abdominal wall defect.

significantly in the last decade, with 1-year and 3-year patient survival improving to 80% and 65%, up from 60% (1 year) and 45% (5 years) previously. However, long-term survival has not improved during this period, with 5-year to 10-year survival less than 50%. The primary cause of death remains sepsis, which has not changed since the inception of intestinal transplantation. Outcomes in children have been reported recently in data from 1987 to 2009, in patients less than 18 years of age (n = 977) (**Table 2**).[19] In this cohort, 1-year, 3-year, and 5-year survival was 85%, 71%, and 65% (for small intestine alone) and 68%, 57%, and 51% (for liver and small intestine combined). Survival for children less than 2 years of age was worse than for all other pediatric age groups. At some high-volume US and European centers, there are recent reports of overall survival as high 84% at 3 years and 77% at 5 years.[2] There are now many patients with more than 20-year survival and there have been reports of successful pregnancies in patients who have had IT. Patient factors associated with higher posttransplant mortality include young patient age (<1 year), hospitalization at the time of transplantation, recipients of isolated intestine or liver-intestine (vs multi-visceral), and nonuse of induction immunosuppression.[20] There seems to be a problem with chronic graft rejection, and an increasing number of long-lived survivors are now requiring retransplantation later in life.

Most IT recipients can be weaned from PN within 1 to 3 months of transplantation. Many of the small children remain on enteral tube feedings for several months after transplantation because they remain unable to take feedings orally because of lack of interest or they have developed complete oral aversion. For this reason, most infants with IF continue to receive oral feedings during infancy, if tolerated, to acquire feeding skills, even if they derive no nutritional benefit. Those children who are fed orally while awaiting IT seem to transition more quickly to oral feedings in the post-transplant period. The optimal formula for tolerance and absorption in the intestinal graft has not been studied in any large-scale, systematic study. Approaches to the advancement of feedings tend to be center specific, but generally begin with elemental peptide formulas. The enteral feedings may be initiated anywhere from the day of transplantation up to 7 days after transplantation. The rate of advancement is also center specific but is generally slow, advancing only 2 to 3 mL/h/d in children. A more immature donor graft may require even slower advancement, given its smaller size and level of physiologic development. Our center has transplanted several children whose mothers have saved breast milk for their children, and we have used this milk in early feedings without complications. The patient is maintained on PN after transplantation to maintain an adequate nutritional level to support healing from the surgery. We maintain full PN support until the enteral feedings have reached

Table 2
Patient survival for pediatric intestine transplantation (1997–2009, n = 977)

Age group (y)	Small Intestine Alone			Small Intestine with Liver		
	1	3	5	1	3	5
<2 y (%)	71	51	41	67	55	51
2–6 y (%)	91	74	71	70	60	53
6–12 y (%)	87	79	71	67	56	53
12–18 y (%)	92	83	74	75	56	56
Overall (%)	85	71	65	68	57	51

Data from Desai CS, Maegawa FB, Gruesner AC, et al. Age-based disparity in outcomes of intestinal transplants in pediatric patients. Am J Transplant 2012;12(Suppl 4):S45; with permission.

one-half of the goal caloric requirements. At this time, we begin to decrease PN on a daily basis, in conjunction with increasing enteral feedings, until the PN is weaned off and full nutritional support is provided through enteral intake. If children are willing to take oral feedings, we allow them to progress at their own rates and decrease PN support accordingly. Nursing staff must be vigilant to record all intake and output to fully monitor graft function and fluid status.

Children are followed closely after transplantation by a multidisciplinary team with close attention to growth and development. However, because of the small number of children with long-term survival, any reports on growth and development result in small case series, which are not well controlled and have limited follow-up. A recent report from the University of California, Los Angeles (UCLA) reports predictors of growth and weight gain in 33 children who underwent IT. With median follow-up of nearly 4 years, most patients were weaned from PN within 30 days of transplantation and maintained normal biochemical parameters for nutrition as well as weight. Patients were noted to have poor catch-up growth, and developed a range of nutritional deficiencies. An earlier article from France reported on 31 children (of 78 patients transplanted during the study period) who had survived at least 2 years after transplantation and were free from PN. Follow-up for this cohort was between 2 and 18 years (median 7 years). Seven patients experienced severe growth failure (23%), with 81% maintaining normal growth velocity up to the time of puberty. Weight was appropriate for height in all cases. There were 5 of 6 patients who achieved normal adult height after puberty, although there was a delay in the onset of puberty. A physiologic study of these children showed fat malabsorption, with normal absorption of proteins and carbohydrates. The researchers suggested that the children in the study engaged in hyperphagia to accommodate the decreased energy absorption of the transplant intestine, and these patients may require 20% to 30% more caloric intake (age adjusted) to maintain growth.[21] Other studies, reporting data from the 1990s, suggest delayed overall growth or had limited follow-up.[22–24]

Posttransplant QOL has been addressed by few/many/several researchers. Common measures for QOL after intestinal transplant include the ability to take oral feedings, organ function, growth and development, and functional measures. In a report by Sudan, and colleagues,[25] from the University of Nebraska, 22 children at a mean age of 11 years (mean follow-up of 5 years) reported similar scores in all QOL measures when compared with age matched peers. The parents of these children, however, noted decreased general health and physical functioning for their child, with a negative effect/affect of the illness on parental time and emotions and family activities. O'Keefe and colleagues,[26] from the University of Pittsburgh, published a QOL report for 38 adult patients who noted a statistically significant improvement in QOL after IT, including improvement in the areas of depression, anxiety, cognitive emotion, appearance, stress, parenting, optimism, control of impulsiveness, medical compliance, relationships, and recreation. A large percentage of these adult patients did not return to full-time employment. In addition, a recent brief report compares the QOL of adult patients on PN with the QOL of those who have undergone IT. Those with IT experience improved QOL across nearly all measures.[27] These limited results suggest that many patients may achieve a good QOL after IT with a well-functioning graft, free of complications. However, there are few data to direct the manner in which these outcomes can be optimized, particularly in children.

COMPLICATIONS AND CONCERNS

Often, patients requiring transplantation of the intestine have required multiple previous surgeries. These surgeries frequently result in extensive scarring, loss of abdominal domain (resulting in a small abdominal cavity), complex anatomy, and chronic pain and narcotic dependence. In addition, chronic malnutrition may lead to poor tissue quality, which increases the risk of anastomotic leak, hernia, poor wound healing, prolonged ventilation, and prolonged hospital stay. Infants and children may also have comorbidities such as chronic infections and congenital anomalies of the heart, lungs, spine, or genitourinary system, which increases the risk of any intervention. When IF is combined with liver cirrhosis and end-stage liver disease, the risks increase even further. One of the indications for intestinal transplantation is loss of vascular access sites. Entering into a transplant procedure with a medically complicated, ill child with limited vascular access risks posttransplant morbidity and mortality. However, options are limited for these children and intestine and multivisceral transplantation stand as a final option for survival.

Surveillance of the intestine graft after transplantation primarily focuses on graft appearance and volume of stool output. Nearly all intestine transplantation procedures provide an ileostomy for easy surveillance of the transplant graft with endoscopy and biopsy. Use of a magnification endoscope is preferable and provides clear visualization of the intestinal villi. Dysmorphic appearance of these villi may be an initial indication of problems, particularly rejection. Monitoring the ostomy for output volume provides an ongoing measure to assess for early complications such as obstruction or rejection. The ostomy output should be consistent, and any extended period of more than 4 to 6 hours without stool output may be cause for concern. When the ostomy output stops, there may be mechanical obstruction, ileus, or overuse of agents that slow motility (such as loperamide, diphenoxylate and atropine, or narcotics such as tincture of opium). Increased output may be related to rejection, infection, medications, malabsorption, or may simply be related to increased enteral intake.

The greatest concern for any patient after IT is for rejection of the graft. With severe rejection of the intestine, there is frequently sloughing of the intestinal mucosa and weakening of the intestinal wall. Unlike solid transplant organs, which are largely sterile, such as the heart, liver, kidney, and pancreas, the intestine contains a heavy load of bacteria in its native state. Therefore, severe rejection and loss of the mucosal barrier can lead to ongoing bacteremia, sepsis, and death. Perforation of the rejecting intestine graft is possible and can be life threatening and require emergent removal of the graft. During rejection, the patient is generally not allowed enteral nutrition and is placed on PN. Recovery from severe rejection can require several weeks to months of increased immunosuppression. However, full recovery is possible and patients can return to normal intestinal function with regrowth of the intestinal mucosa. Severe rejection may be associated with fibrosis and scarring, which affects long-term intestinal function and may be related to symptoms of chronic rejection. In a clinical scenario of severe rejection with ongoing complications, the decision is often taken to remove the transplant graft. With the graft removed, the immunosuppression can be stopped. The patient may then recover and be transplanted again at a later date. Simultaneous transplantation of the small intestine with the liver seems to protect against rejection in the intestine. This tolerogenic effect of the liver has been described in other combination transplants and its immunologic basis is not understood.

Because of the potentially devastating effects of rejection, patients who have had IT are almost universally overimmunosuppressed in the early posttransplant period. This overimmunosuppression leads to a high rate of infections, and the leading cause of death is sepsis. Infectious sources are varied, but include typical species and sites including blood stream, urine, the wound, and the respiratory system. In a report of pediatric patients who had had IT at the University of Miami, Florida, the infection rate was 91%, with a median of 5 infections per child.[20] Antibiotic coverage in the posttransplantation period is broad, and empiric therapy can continue for days or weeks, depending on patient progress. Prophylactic coverage for cytomegalovirus, *Pneumocystis jiroveci*, and fungus is mandatory, often for at least 1 year after transplantation. Other immunologic-related complications common in intestine transplantation are posttransplant lymphoproliferative disorder and graft-versus-host disease (GVHD). These diseases processes frequently respond to therapy, but can be life threatening when they are nonresponsive.

As with other transplants, renal toxicity is a common complication related to the chronic use of the calcineurin inhibitors, either tacrolimus or cyclosporine. This toxicity is more significant in intestine transplant patients because of the higher serum levels required in these patients to prevent rejection. Efforts have been made to minimize this damage through the early use of antibody-based immunosuppression induction, with an expectation that lower serum levels of the calcineurin inhibitors will be required in the early posttransplant period. Use of these agents, primarily rabbit antithymocyte globulin (rATG or thymoglobulin) or alemtuzumab, is now ubiquitous at all intestine transplant programs, with some adding basiliximab. Over time, a level of tolerance seems to occur because many patients can be managed with lower levels of calcineurin inhibitor or changed to another agent with less renal toxicity, such as sirolimus.

SUMMARY

A large number of infants and small children are left dependent on long-term PN as a result of a variety of complications including NEC, gastroschisis, malrotation, volvulus, and other congenital anomalies. PN is associated with a variety of complications including frequent central venous catheter infections, loss of vascular access, electrolyte and fluid derangements, and cholestatic liver disease. Every effort should be made through intestinal rehabilitation to minimize these complications and to wean these children from PN to enteral feedings, and eventually to an oral diet. Some of these children will fail available medical and surgical therapy. For these children, IT offers the chance for a return to enteral autonomy, and normal growth and development. Children with ultrashort gut, full-length Hirschsprung disease, or other nontreatable diseases or enteropathies may be identified early as poor candidates for intestinal rehabilitation. These children should be referred early for intestinal transplantation to avoid the complications and nutritional and physiologic deterioration that can occur with long-term PN. Those children who are candidates for rehabilitation must be monitored closely for the development of life-threatening complications that may preclude candidacy for later IT should they fail rehabilitation.

IT in children has evolved to one of 2 procedures, isolated transplantation of the small intestine in children with normal liver function, or liver/small intestine (or multivisceral) transplantation in children with irreversible liver fibrosis or cirrhosis. The wait-list time for an isolated small intestine graft is short, whereas the surgical procedure is less complex. For children awaiting simultaneous small intestine and liver transplantation, the clinical situation may be dire. These children are put into the pool of all children awaiting liver transplantation, with its accompanying long wait-list time. The longer wait-list time results in further ongoing risk for catheter infections and episodes of sepsis, loss of vascular access, and dehydration and electrolyte abnormalities. The liver disease continues to progress as the child still requires daily PN for survival. When the donor organs become available, the surgical transplant is more complex, and the child is often more debilitated compared with a child without end-stage liver disease. This complexity increases the risk for operative and perioperative morbidity and mortality.

Clinical outcomes for IT have been mixed. In recent years, the risk of dying while awaiting transplantation has decreased. Children at risk are now more likely to be identified early and referred to a center with expertise in IF. From there, they receive appropriate interventions and are more likely to be referred for IT if they meet criteria. Early posttransplantation outcomes have improved. More patients are referred for IT before the onset of severe debilitation, and their ability to withstand the IT procedure and recovery period has improved. Transplant surgical technique and postoperative intensive care unit management has improved. Also, immunosuppression therapy has improved. With the advent of antibody-based immunosuppression induction, used in conjunction with tacrolimus-based maintenance therapy, there is less early rejection. However, the long-term outcomes are largely unchanged. The development of chronic rejection several years after transplantation is common and often results in the need for retransplantation. There are a large number of infections in patients who have had IT, and certain neoplasms and GVHD are more common in patients who have had IT patient compared with recipients of other transplant organs. There are many 10-year to 20-year survivors with good QOL, and these patients must be analyzed to identify the best candidates for the transplant option. Recipients of an uncomplicated IT report a much improved QOL, and children with successful IT are likely to experience normal growth and development.

The history of transplantation provides hope for continued advancement. The development of transplantation of each of the individual solid organs (heart, lung, kidney, liver, and pancreas) has followed a sometimes troubled path to reach routine success. Intestinal transplantation seems to be on that same trajectory and provides a reasonable hope for patients with IF with a terminal disease and no other options.

REFERENCES

1. Squires RH, Duggan C, Teitelbaum DH. Natural history of pediatric intestinal failure: initial report from the pediatric intestinal failure consortium. J Pediatr 2012;161(4):723–728.e2.
2. Mazariegos GV, Superina R, Rudolph J, et al. Current status of pediatric intestinal failure, rehabilitation, and transplantation: summary of a colloquium. Transplantation 2011;92(11):1173.
3. Avitzur Y, Grant D. Intestine transplantation in children: update 2010. Pediatr Clin North Am 2010;57(2):415.
4. Goulet O. The Second World Congress of Pediatric Gastroenterology, Hepatology and Nutrition: Paris, 3–7 July 2004. J Pediatr Gastroenterol Nutr 2004; 38(1):1.
5. Goulet O, Ruemmele F, Lacaille F, et al. Irreversible intestinal failure. J Pediatr Gastroenterol Nutr 2004;38(3):250.
6. Sondheimer JM, Cadnapaphornchai M, Sontag M, et al. Predicting the duration of dependence on parenteral nutrition after neonatal intestinal resection. J Pediatr 1998;132(1):80.
7. Beath S, Pironi L, Gabe S, et al. Collaborative strategies to reduce mortality and morbidity in patients with chronic intestinal failure including those who are referred for small bowel transplantation. Transplantation 2008;85(10):1378.
8. Struijs MC, Sloots CJ, Tibboel D. The gap in referral criteria for pediatric intestinal transplantation. Transplantation 2012;94:92.
9. Lopushinsky SR, Fowler RA, Kulkarni GS, et al. The optimal timing of intestinal transplantation for children with intestinal failure: a Markov analysis. Ann Surg 2007;246(6):1092.

10. Diamond IR, Sterescu A, Pencharz PB, et al. Changing the paradigm: Omegaven for the treatment of liver failure in pediatric short bowel syndrome. J Pediatr Gastroenterol Nutr 2009;48(2):209.

11. Gura KM, Duggan CP, Collier SB, et al. Reversal of parenteral nutrition-associated liver disease in two infants with short bowel syndrome using parenteral fish oil: implications for future management. Pediatrics 2006;118(1):e197.

12. Cowles RA, Ventura KA, Martinez M, et al. Reversal of intestinal failure-associated liver disease in infants and children on parenteral nutrition: experience with 93 patients at a referral center for intestinal rehabilitation. J Pediatr Surg 2010; 45(1):84.

13. Oliveira C, Nasr A, Brindle M, et al. Ethanol locks to prevent catheter-related bloodstream infections in parenteral nutrition: a meta-analysis. Pediatrics 2012; 129(2):318.

14. Hess RA, Welch KB, Brown PI, et al. Survival outcomes of pediatric intestinal failure patients: analysis of factors contributing to improved survival over the past two decades. J Surg Res 2011;170(1):27.

15. Sudan D. Advances in the nontransplant medical and surgical management of intestinal failure. Curr Opin Organ Transplant 2009;14(3):274.

16. Carlsen BT, Farmer DG, Busuttil RW, et al. Incidence and management of abdominal wall defects after intestinal and multivisceral transplantation. Plast Reconstr Surg 2007;119(4):1247.

17. Gondolesi G, Selvaggi G, Tzakis A, et al. Use of the abdominal rectus fascia as a nonvascularized allograft for abdominal wall closure after liver, intestinal, and multivisceral transplantation. Transplantation 2009;87(12):1884.

18. Mangus RŚ, Kubal CA, Tector AJ, et al. Closure of the abdominal wall with acellular dermal allograft in intestinal transplantation. Am J Transplant 2012; 12(Suppl 4):S55–9.

19. Desai CS, Maegawa FB, Gruesner AC, et al. Age-based disparity in outcomes of intestinal transplants in pediatric patients. Am J Transplant 2012;12(Suppl 4): S43–8.

20. Kato T, Tzakis AG, Selvaggi G, et al. Intestinal and multivisceral transplantation in children. Ann Surg 2006;243(6):756.

21. Lacaille F, Vass N, Sauvat F, et al. Long-term outcome, growth and digestive function in children 2 to 18 years after intestinal transplantation. Gut 2008;57(4):455.

22. Iyer K, Horslen S, Iverson A, et al. Nutritional outcome and growth of children after intestinal transplantation. J Pediatr Surg 2002;37(3):464.

23. Encinas JL, Luis A, Avila LF, et al. Nutritional status after intestinal transplantation in children. Eur J Pediatr Surg 2006;16(6):403.

24. Nucci AM, Barksdale EM Jr, Beserock N, et al. Long-term nutritional outcome after pediatric intestinal transplantation. J Pediatr Surg 2002;37(3):460.

25. Sudan D, Horslen S, Botha J, et al. Quality of life after pediatric intestinal transplantation: the perception of pediatric recipients and their parents. Am J Transplant 2004;4(3):407.

26. O'Keefe SJ, Emerling M, Koritsky D, et al. Nutrition and quality of life following small intestinal transplantation. Am J Gastroenterol 2007;102(5):1093.

27. Pironi LB, Lauro JP, Guidetti A, et al. Assessment of quality of life on home parenteral nutrition and after intestinal transplantation using treatment-specific questionnaires. Am J Transplant 2012;12(Suppl 4):S60–6.

Index

Note: Page numbers of article titles are in **boldface** type.

A

Abdominal signs, 33–35
Absorbent agents, for short bowel syndrome, 62
Acid suppression, for short bowel syndrome, 61
Acute-phase proteins, 153
Adaptation, in short bowel syndrome, 55–56
Advancement, of feeding, 4–5
Amyloid, 153–154
Anastomosis, with bowel resection, 141–142
Anastomotic ulcers, 144
Anoikis, in lactoferrin action, 83–84
Anomalies, with necrotizing enterocolitis, 28
Antibiotics
    for NEC, 38–39, 138
    for short bowel syndrome, 58–59
    microbiota population and, 101–102
Anti-diarrheal agents, for short bowel syndrome, 62
Anti-inflammatory mechanisms, of lactoferrin, 82
Apple-peel intestinal atresia, 55
Ascites, 137

B

Bacterial overgrowth, in short bowel syndrome, 58
Bacteroides, colonization by, 13
Bell classification, of NEC, 138
Bifidobacteria
    colonization by, 13, 32
    in probiotic formulations, 14
    metabolomics of, 98
    outcomes of, 17–18
    prebiotics for, 15
Billard, Charles, 27–28
Biomarkers, 127–128, **149–159**
    genetic, 128, 150–152
    metagenomics of, 152
    nonspecific, 153–154
    novel, 155–156
    of oxidative stress, 152
    predictive value of, 150–152
    specific, 154–155
Blood transfusions, 31

Clin Perinatol 40 (2013) 175–183
http://dx.doi.org/10.1016/S0095-5108(13)00013-4
0095-5108/13/$ – see front matter © 2013 Elsevier Inc. All rights reserved.
perinatology.theclinics.com

Moving?

Make sure your subscription moves with you!

To notify us of your new address, find your **Clinics Account Number** (located on your mailing label above your name), and contact customer service at:

Email: journalscustomerservice-usa@elsevier.com

800-654-2452 (subscribers in the U.S. & Canada)
314-447-8871 (subscribers outside of the U.S. & Canada)

Fax number: 314-447-8029

Elsevier Health Sciences Division
Subscription Customer Service
3251 Riverport Lane
Maryland Heights, MO 63043

ELSEVIER